MW01233266

THE
ESTHETICIAN'S
GUIDE TO
OUTSTANDING
ESTHETICS!
VOL II

Technical Know-How from Today's Industry Icons

Anthology Compiled By:

SHELLEY HANCOCK

Licensed Esthetician Since 1988

Skin Care Center Owner Since 1990

DEDICATION

This book is dedicated to all of my fellow Estheticians that aspire
to bring outstanding esthetics to their clients. We hope to inspire
you with our stories of success and let you know
that all things are possible.

I'd like to thank my husband for being right beside me
and always encouraging me to jump.
Love you!

TABLE OF CONTENTS

Introduction

The Estheticians Guide to Outstanding Esthetics Volume II Technical Know-How from Today's Industry Icons is the second book in a series of Anthology books for the beauty industry. I decided to publish this series of books because the esthetic industry was in need of inspiration (volume I) as well as technical information (volume II) from its leaders. These industry leaders are the cream of the crop and were chosen to author a chapter which provides technical information in different aspects of the industry so that you can achieve outstanding results in your esthetic career and/or your spa business.

When I titled this book Outstanding Esthetics, I knew I was raising the bar. Outstanding Esthetics can mean many things but at the end of the day, achieving something that is outstanding takes a lot of time and hard work. Sometimes we don't want to put in the hard work it takes to achieve outstanding results, or we don't know how to get there, or perhaps there are too many obstacles in our way. If you are experiencing this then start reading.

There are a couple of ways to read this book. You can read it cover to cover or pick and choose the chapters that most interest you and read just those. I highly recommend reading every chapter as all the information in this book is invaluable. Either way, I know you will walk away with the advice and know-how you need to move your esthetic career in the right direction . . . forward toward success.

This book is abounding with helpful information. Therefore, I suggest you get out your highlighter, dog ear your favorite pages, take notes with paper and pen, or on your device. You'll want to keep track of all your newly found tips and ideas that will shape and change your esthetic world. There will be many nuggets you can use; I guarantee that!

I know myself, and the authors of the Outstanding Esthetics book series welcome your thoughts and comments. I urge you to reach out to any specific author who really made you think or provided you with new information. Send an email to let them know your thoughts or provide some comments. I know all of us will appreciate your insights as to what moved you, changed you, and got you to the results you deserve.

Thank you for letting us help you on your results-oriented journey to greater success in the world of esthetics.

Much love…Shelley Hancock

Shelley Hancock

Chapter 1

Cutting Edge Esthetic Equipment

Authored by Shelley Hancock

In September 2018, I'll be celebrating 30 years as an esthetician and 29 years as a skincare business owner. Here's what I know for sure: to create and sustain a successful skin care business, we need to stay up with the ever growing and changing esthetic equipment technology. Today's clients are savvy and results-oriented. There is so much information readily available to them on the Internet. They are investigating these technologies and they want to know that we are up on them as well. No longer are they satisfied with a good old-fashioned steam facial. Fortunately for us, we have the equipment to achieve the kind of results they're looking for.

I've been following the ever-changing technologies throughout the years, testing just about every new modality that has shown up. I can remember back when you were considered high tech if your steamer had aromatherapy! Things have changed and now we can truly offer our clients cutting edge, results-oriented treatments.

When you offer treatments using high-tech equipment that achieve immediate results, your clients will be your walking advertisements. Their friends will see those results and inquire what they're up to and with whom. Now you've got loyal, lifetime clients and instant referrals.

Let's chat about some of the modalities and what role they play in your facial treatments...

Exfoliation: What's the first thing that to comes to mind when asked about equipment for exfoliation? Microdermabrasion, right? It was really the only modality around in the 90's. So, all clients got a microderm treatment whether they needed it or not. To boost the intensity, we topped it off with an acid peel. Today, I like to use the DermaDisc Exfoliator. It achieves the same great exfoliation as the diamond microdermabrasion machine but with no suction. For details about mechanical exfoliation, read the chapter by Mary Neilson.

How about ultrasound for exfoliation? I believe it's a must-have in every esthetic tool box. Using sound waves of 25,000 to 28,000 vibrations per second is most effective for exfoliation. I use the Ultrasonic Spatula in every treatment. I do not consider using this tool as an add-on. I use it to take off my cleanser (now, you have a deep cleanse) and I also use it to take off all my enzymes. Complete details about ultrasound are found in the chapter by Beatrice Van.

The "big guns" of equipment for exfoliation is the OxyGeneo. This is a newer technology to our industry. Not only does it exfoliate, but it oxygenates from within too. It capitalizes on the Bohr Effect that was discovered by Christian Bohr in 1904. This effect indicates that when carbon dioxide concentrations increase, the hemoglobin releases oxygen from within. The interaction between the special capsugen tablet and the treatment gel on the skin creates an abundance of CO_2 that triggers the Bohr Effect, thus oxygenating the skin from within. This reaction is also exfoliating. These effects are beneficial in anti-aging, re-texturizing, and correcting pigmentation issues. Powerful exfoliation with no irritation. You can't beat that!

Hydration: What tools are used for deep product penetration and hydrating the skin? Ultrasound, right? The sound waves act on the body in the following way: they stimulate cells. The tiny massage they produce stimulate and expand the cell membrane by causing movement of cytoplasm, rotation of mitochondria, and vibration of the cell nucleus. It improves local blood and lymph circulation, and increases the penetration of the fabulous products you are using in treatment. Again, read the chapter by Beatrice Van for complete details.

Another hydrating modality is electroporation. This modality uses short modulated pulses of high voltage to create transient aqueous pores in the skin. This application of an electrical pulse momentarily disrupts the cell membrane allowing the entry of product. When the pulse ceases, the membrane returns to its original structure, leaving product that has penetrated into the interior of the cell in place. The effect of the electroporation lasts for a few seconds, therefore, allowing the introduction of product into the cell. In simple language, electroporation opens a door (or pathway) that allows us to insert products deeper into the skin.

Another interesting hydrating modality is HIFU or High Intensity Focused Ultrasound. High energy ultrasound, focused directly where the unit is positioned on the face, creates a thermal effect that in turn creates high-speed friction within the cells to stimulate collagen and elastin. This heat will not affect the epidermis because of the fast (about a half a second) and direct access to the area being treated. I am really liking this modality not only for hydration, but for some toning as well!

The Rezenerate is another fabulous piece of equipment for hydrating the skin. Rezenerate utilizes the breakthrough science of Nano-Technology and a proprietary process to create what they have dubbed the "Rezenerate Nano-Tech Golden Ratio." It delivers consistent results time and time again. I've even seen toning on the jawline of one of my clients and I truly wasn't expecting that! Read the chapter by Ryan Rabah for full details.

Brightening: I love LED for brightening up the skin. I've been using it since 2002. At my Center, LED is included in every treatment we offer. All clients get a minimum of 10 minutes under the LED panel at the end of their treatments. I just factor it into the time and cost. LED can be used with all skin issues (anti-aging, acne, rosacea, pigmentation, etc.) and all skin types.

Another light-based technology is MicroPhototherapy. Using the healing power of LHE (light and heat energy) to stimulate faster production of collagen and elastin, MicroPhototherapy allows new fresh cells to surface, which brightens the skin. This is the best modality that I have found for pigmentation issues. I've been using this modality for over 8 years and it's still one of my favorite treatments. It's definitely the WOW factor.

Oxygen Infusion is another brightening and super hydrating treatment. This is one of those treatments that clients thoroughly enjoy. It offers instant gratification. The sensation is refreshing and relaxing. Once your client has experienced a quality oxygen infusion treatment, they will always want it included in their facial. It's great for deep hydration and plumping fine lines, and depending on the product you are infusing you can help other issues such as pigmentation and acne.

Toning: Microcurrent is the well-known modality in our industry for toning and tightening. Tiny microcurrent impulses trigger chemical reactions at a cellular level, working directly on nerves and muscle fibers to enhance the production of natural collagen and elastin and provide circulatory benefits. Your body seems to use the microcurrent energy to increase its own energy production, resulting in visible firming and smoothing of the skin. Here's what I truly believe about microcurrent…you need very good training to do a proper treatment and many machines come with little or no training. It's very technical and needs to be done properly to achieve optimum results. Read the chapter by Tina Abnoosi for details.

The OxyGeneo that I spoke of earlier also offers a toning effect. They call it the Three-in-One Super Facial. The first step is exfoliation/oxygenation, the second step is ultrasound for deep hydration, and the third is a high-level vibration hand piece that I believe kicks in the toning effect.

Another modality that I used quite a lot in the 90's is High Frequency. I got away from it for many years and have just connected with it again. I mainly used it for acne back in the day, but I've opened to the idea of using it for anti-aging. I must tell you, it works! When mixed with the air outside of the unit, the electrical current infuses the skin with rejuvenating oxygen molecules, which causes a circulation rush. Your skin just feels awake after using high frequency. I wasn't sure which category to place this modality in because it hydrates, brightens, and kills bacteria.

That sums up some of the effective tools we can use in treatment to achieve results that keep our clients coming back for more.

It's a fabulous industry we have chosen to be a part of. Keep yourself educated and you will prosper. But most important, enjoy your work every day because people are drawn to that positive energy!

About Shelley Hancock

Shelley Hancock, (a.k.a 'The Gadget Gal'), is one of the most trusted esthetic advisors of our time and Founder of Shelley Hancock Consulting, an organization dedicated to helping estheticians increase their profits. After owning a successful skin care center for 29 years, Hancock expanded her focus so she could provide a deeper level of service to fellow estheticians. Through hands-on training, workshops and private consultations, she has now connected 1000s of beauty business owners with esthetic equipment that attracts a higher level client and helps build a more successful practice. "Most retailers think the relationship ends with purchase," explains Hancock. "I view it as just the beginning".

When she's not teaching, training, coaching or working with clients, you will find her recording her radio program for Voice America.

Contact Shelley Today!

Website: http://www.ShelleyHancock.com

Email: contactme@shelleyhancock.com

Chapter 2

Integrative Esthetics

Authored by Becky Kuehn
Founder, Oncology Spa Solutions®, creator of the Life Changing Esthetics® and the MBA (Mindfulness-Based Aesthetics) programs for Spa Professionals

Integrative Esthetics is a combination of Esthetics with other modalities used holistically to treat or care for clients. There are many of them, but I am going to share with you the joyous wonders of implementing *mindfulness* into our treatment rooms. It will change your business (and your life)!

A student shared an experience with me regarding mindfulness that I would like to share with you. A new client booked a facial and upon arriving, the Esthetician sensed a heavy, depressed, sad energy. Now, the Esthetician could have been turned off or scared (both are totally normal reactions) but instead, she chose a different approach. She decided to mindfully engage and take it on as a challenge. She envisioned the energy as something "physical" that she could "move", not just out of her client, but out of the room and into the heavens (kind of like a symphony conductor). As she began her treatment, she silently said a little prayer, and kept good, positive thoughts in her head throughout the treatment while visualizing the heavy energy being moved, lifted, and removed from the room.

OK...it may sound weird to you, or as my husband would say, it may sound a little "woo woo". Chances are, YOU have experienced something like this. Because we are all made up of energy, this happens *every time* we encounter another human being. And we can train ourselves to take notice.

The end of the story truly impacted me. The client loved her treatment, thanked the Esty, said she felt fabulous and had never experienced anything like it, and left. Then a week later, the client's daughter contacted the Esthetician to share the "back story". She explained that her mom had lost her husband some months prior and had been so depressed and sad that she wore black every day since. After the treatment, her mom was a whole new person and even started wearing colors again. The daughter wanted to know: "WHAT in the world had the Esthetician done to make such a difference?" (oh, and the mom became a regular, the daughter became a client, and several others from their circle became clients as well).

Sometimes, I think as Estheticians we take for granted or are unaware of the gift and power we hold regarding the simple but profound act of touch. Did you know that Estheticians are one of the very few professionals who are licensed to touch another human being? And we get to do it every day. The unfortunate part is that we learned the steps to our facial so long ago and some have never varied far from that original protocol. In fact, we know it so well that we (can) easily fall into what I call "Esty autopilot". You know what I mean...being able to do a facial blindfolded without even thinking about each individual step. When we are on autopilot, are we really *with* our client? Do you "go through the motions" of your facial while thinking about something else (grocery shopping, dinner, relationship issues, etc.)? As part of the Oncology Spa Solutions® training, we try to tackle this problem. We invite cancer patients/survivors to come in and share their journeys with us. Then, the students develop and provide customized treatments to meet their unique needs. Afterwards, I ask the clients to share what the experience was like or what it meant to them. Most times, the answer is: "Wow, I loved it, thank you for what you are doing, for hearing our needs, and being here for us." Occasionally, they feel like a student was "not there". That breaks my heart. I firmly believe that all clients should receive the care and attention they need and deserve; they should get our very best. This is important for cancer patients, but for healthy clients too. Also, an incredible moment for the Esty is lost. These Estheticians are missing out on the richness and personal reward of connecting with another soul. My goal and passion is to change that in our industry. I had a client one time at the hospital tell me that she was so excited for our time together that she marked it on her calendar and counted down the days until her appointment. What if I didn't feel like worki

day? What if I showed up physically but was not there for her

mindfully?

I found it quite interesting that while researching energy, touch, and mindfulness I came across many articles regarding dogs. Yes, dogs! A dear friend who is a dog trainer once told me: "you don't have to say a word to your dog, your feelings travel through the leash." So if our dog can feel our energy without us saying a word or touching them, how much more aware are our clients? Dogs, by the way, are WAY ahead of us when it comes to mindfulness. They live in the present moment every day with integrity, loyalty, and love. We can learn many lessons from them as they are *naturally* more aware than humans... *We* need to *learn* and *practice* *mindfulness* before it becomes a natural response.

So, let's dig a little into "mindfulness", define its meaning, and discuss how to use it in a practical way.

Even though "mindfulness" is NOT a new word, it gets used a lot these days, especially in our industry. Scarcely used since its inception in the early 1500's, mindfulness became more understood, recognized, and popular in the 1950's.

Definitions of Mindfulness:

- "The practice of maintaining a nonjudgmental state of heightened or complete awareness of one's thoughts, emotions, or experiences on a moment-to-moment basis." (Merriam-Webster)

- "The practice of being aware of your body, mind, and feelings in the present moment, thought to create a feeling of calm." (Cambridge Dictionary)

- "Mindfulness is about observation without criticism; being compassionate with yourself." (Mindfulness: Finding Peace in a Frantic World)

- "Mindfulness is the aware, balanced acceptance of the present experience. It isn't more complicated than that. It is opening to or receiving the present moment, pleasant or unpleasant, just as it is, without either clinging to it or rejecting it." (Sylvia Boorstein)

- "Mindfulness is learning to be open and receptive for every moment and experience of our lives; paying attention to our surroundings and connecting with those in our path". (Becky Kuehn)

Using Mindfulness-Based Aesthetics in the treatment room:

- **Connect with your clients during intake/consent** – sit across from them without anything in between. Sit close and make eye contact when you are asking questions or explaining the treatment.

- **Be real and share yourself with your clients** – that means being open, listening wholeheartedly, using touch with intention, and being your authentic self. Visualize your energy, compassion, and love flowing through your hands. (This does not mean talking about yourself).

- **Listen to and meet the needs/concerns of your clients** – How do you know what their needs are? Ask! And then – surpass their expectations! One of the most common client/customer complaints is that they did not get what they came in for. Oncology clients think "no one listens to me." So, one little (but BIG) thing we could add to our practice is communication with intention and focus on our client. This will make a difference in client satisfaction and re-booking, which will increase your business.

- **Take a minute to read the consent form and come up with a plan** – this step gets missed quite often and it's VERY important! In the OSS training, we teach the **CAT** method. **CAT** stands for: **Consult** – take all the information. **Analyze** – read it, know it so that you listen to your clients' needs. **Treat** – now come up with custom treatment plans specific to them.

- **Dimmed lights, soft music, slightly warm bed and a wonderful, soft aroma** – these things matter. They might seem like little things, but as they say, "it's the little things that make ALL the difference." (Tip: Choose soft and slow music without words *IF* you want your clients to relax. As for the aroma – put 1 drop of an Essential oil blend for relaxing the nervous system on a cotton round in your hot towel cabby. It will be soft, warm, and not overwhelming).

- **Before you start, take a big, deep breath** – slowly in through your nose and out through your mouth. Clear your thoughts, clear your mind, and set your intentions on your clients' needs. Depending on your mindfulness level, you might have to take two or three breaths. (Tip: Have your client breathe with you, which will relax them and set the stage).

- **Now you are ready to place your hands on your client and let the magic begin-** move slowly and with intention. I guarantee it will make a difference.

Love others, love what you do and the world will take notice!

ooxx

Becky

About Becky Kuehn

Becky is the passionate founder of Oncology Spa Solutions®. Her mission, along with her team of angel trainers, is to share with others how to care for clients when they have cancer, how to connect with Dr's, and how to make a difference in their communities.

Join her in changing lives!

Contact Becky Today!

Website: http://www.oncologyspasolutions.com
Email: Becky@oncologyspasolutions.com

Chapter 3

Chemical Exfoliation

Authored by Mary Nielsen

Chemical peels are very useful in an aesthetician's tool box and work well when integrated into a full treatment plan for a client. Chemical peels, a form of chemical exfoliation, are categorized according to strength. There are four strengths of chemical peels understood in the aesthetic realm: very superficial, superficial, medium depth, and deep. Each category has a specific depth that the chemicals can penetrate the skin. In addition, each category usually has an associated pH or strength.

What influences a peel more than its ingredients is its pH. This measurement determines the strength of the peel. The pH of the skin is 5.5, which is slightly acidic. Anything below a 5.5 pH is categorized as an acid, which will irritate or burn. Anything above a 5.5 pH is categorized as an alkali or base, which can also be irritating but an alkali is not as predictable or reliable as an acid. Therefore, all chemical peels are acids. Burning creates an injury to the tissue. It is in the healing process that the benefits of the peel are reached.

A brief overview of the peel categories follows, as well as information on peel ingredients.

Very superficial peels are mild exfoliants. The client's skin is cleansed and the chemical solution is applied. Clients may experience a slight stinging sensation or they may experience nothing. There is little to no down time with a very superficial peel because the skin may peel microscopically, with very little visible shedding. Risks are minimal with a very superficial peel. A very superficial peel is a good option because it can be used safely on all skin types. It can enhance collagen production and smooth the skin's texture. It allows skin care products to penetrate more evenly, so it is a great option for skin polishing before a spray tan or to create more luminosity in the skin before a big event.

A superficial peel is the most common type of peel that aestheticians apply. This type of peel works no deeper than the epidermis, with ingredients ranging up to 30 percent with a pH greater than 3.0. There can be visible peeling; a slight shedding that begins about 48 hours after the peel is applied. Superficial peels are best done in a series of increasing ingredient strength; one peel every four to six weeks. The peel can strengthen the dermis, create collagen, treat sun-damaged skin, and reduce fine lines. Superficial peels cannot tighten skin laxity.

A medium depth peel works at the papillary-reticular dermal junction and has a pH below 3.0. It will create some strong shedding that can last for a week, starting about 48 hours after the peel is applied. A medium depth peel improves skin texture, fine lines, sun damage and will continue to build collagen for six to twelve months after the peel.

Deep chemical peels are best left to skilled medical professionals.

These peels contain toxic ingredients that can cause cardiac arrest if not done properly. They are extremely painful and usually done in conjunction with a facelift while the client is under anesthesia. The down time is equally dramatic. A person may have one or two deep chemical peels in a lifetime.

Some common enzyme peel ingredients come from fruits. Papain is from papaya. Bromelain comes from pineapple. Actinidin is from kiwi. Pumpkin peels are another common enzyme peel. Enzyme peels are effective because the enzyme eats away and dissolves the bonds between dead skin cells.

Some common acid peels include alpha hydroxy acids (AHAs), beta hydroxy acids (BHA), trichloroacetic acids (TCA), and cocktailed peels.

Alpha hydroxy acids are derived mostly from fruit acids or dairy. They are typically safe for most skin types. They are water soluble, meaning they are attracted to the water in the skin. The pH of the AHA peel causes a 'shock' to the skin cells and loosens the bonds of the desmosomes, the glue that holds the stratum corneum's dead skin cells together. Alpha hydroxy acid peels must be neutralized with either water or a sodium bicarbonate solution.

Glycolic acids come from sugar cane. They are usually best done in a series of increasing strength. Glycolic acid is the smallest molecule of the alpha hydroxy acids so it penetrates well. Glycolic acids are best used for improving photo damaged skin, improving fine lines and rough texture, as well as improving skin elasticity as it builds collagen.

Lactic acid derives from sour milk. It works well on rosacea and sensitive skin. It also helps with dry skin, which may seem counterintuitive. Lactic acid creates low TEWL, or Trans-Epidermal Water Loss. It allows moisture to evaporate more slowly off the skin. It works well for acne skin, sun damage, and reducing the appearance of large pores.

Other alpha hydroxy acids include citric acid from citrus fruits, tartaric acid from grapes, and malic acid from pears and apples.

Salicylic acid is the best-known beta hydroxy acid, or BHA. It is found in willow bark and manufactured synthetically. It is lipid soluble, so it is attracted to the oil in the skin. It breaks up the oil and is very good for sebaceous follicle blockage. It is antimicrobial so it's a great choice for treating acne. It is self-neutralizing. Clients may experience a 'false' frost, or a frosting on the skin due to the evaporation of solution, leaving behind the salicylic crystals. Salicylic acid can be toxic so should not be applied to more than 20 percent of the body during a peel session.

Trichloroacetic acid is a widely-used peel, often mixed with other ingredients. The client will experience a deep heating sensation with this peel. It is self-neutralizing. TCA will frost upon application as the protein in the skin coagulates in response to the chemical reaction taking place.

Cocktailed peels hit the market in the early 2000s and their popularity has increased each year as new options open for a transformational skin rejuvenation. Several acids, including TCA (trichloroacetic acid), AHA, BHA, phenol, and resorcinol, are blended in small percentages with vitamin C, retinol, and other additives that infuse the skin with healing and repairing while sloughing off the dead layers.

Many of these cocktailed peels have boosters like kojic acid, hydroquinone, or others that allow the aesthetician to tailor the peel to specific skin conditions, such as hyper-pigmentation of melasma or acne breakouts.

It is imperative that the aesthetician double checks client allergies. Clients who have allergies to specific foods should not have a peel with those ingredients. This includes an allergy to Aspirin when considering a salicylic peel, as both Aspirin and salicylic come from the same salicylate compounds.

Client Consultation: The intention of a consultation is to interview the client and find out how much down time, even if it's social downtime, she or he is willing to accept after a peel. This will help the practitioner determine if a series of superficial peels or a medium depth peel with more aggressive peeling would be best. It is a disaster to find out during peel application that the client will be the mother-of-the-bride during the timeframe she will experience the heaviest peeling!

Indications and Contraindications: Indications for a peel are varied and will include an assessment of the client's skin condition and appropriate peel for that skin condition. Photo rejuvenation, an improvement in fine lines and texture, reduction in acneic breakouts, and improvement in rosacea breakouts are all realistic expectations after a chemical peel.

Treatment: The client should sign an informed consent form for treatment. Expectations should be reviewed and the client should have the opportunity to ask questions. Photos should be taken pre-treatment. With gloves on, you should cleanse the skin thoroughly and use a degreasing agent to remove any oils from the skin that will impede penetration of the peel solution. Some peels come with a prepping solution but isopropyl alcohol, acetone, and which hazel are some options that may be used.

Apply a barrier of petrolatum to the corners of the client's eyes, mouth, and nose.

Have a bowl of tepid water, compresses, or 4x4 gauze on hand. A 10cc syringe filled with normal saline should be available in case peel solution creeps into the client's eyes. It can be used for immediately irrigating the eye and rinsing out the peel solution.

Instruct the client to close his/her eyes. While wearing gloves, use a 2x2 gauze to apply the peel. Begin at the outer perimeter of the face and move toward the center. Apply with even pressure and quick motions. Reinforce application in the client's troubled areas. Watch for pooling of the peel solution in the corners of the nose or crow's feet. Use a timer to time how long the peel solution is on the face. The peel should be applied for the amount of time or the clinical endpoint indicated by the manufacturer, unless the client reports feeling discomfort at a level above seven on a scale of 1–10. If the client reports extreme discomfort, the peel should be neutralized with the neutralizing solution or water immediately.

If frosting is an endpoint, the skin must be closely observed. The number of layers applied to the skin is determined by the manufacturer. If visible frosting is evident, additional layers should not be applied. A light frost with a pink background indicates the peel has penetrated to the papillary dermis. Apply the neutralizing solution followed by cool compresses until the stinging sensation from the peel application dissipates, which is when the peel time limit has been met. It is not unusual to require cool compresses for ten minutes or more.

Apply a hydrating serum or moisturizer and a mineral-based SPF.

When performing a chemical peel on a non-facial part of the body, it's important to understand that the face heals more predictably and faster than the body. The chest and neck will require more healing time.

Side Effects and Complications: The client should feel some itching or tingling during the treatment. Mild erythema and skin sensitivity following the peel is common. Peeling should occur two days after the peel, if peeling is appropriate. Some very superficial peels will not cause visible peeling. The client's skin may feel sunburned.

Mild to moderate edema may occur and the client may want to sleep with his/her head elevated.

Hyper-pigmentation is a complication with darker Fitzpatrick skin types, and should resolve within six months. However, it may be permanent so peel selection and application are very important.

Post Treatment: The client must keep his/her skin moist with moisturizer and SPF. The client should avoid heat inducing activity, like heavy exercise, for 48 hours after a peel. The client can resume a skin care regimen once peeling is completed, usually around 5 to 7 days after the peel. Clients avoid sun exposure for several weeks due to sensitivity.

Documentation: Documentation should include the client's skin condition pre-treatment, the type of peel solution used, the degreasing agent, the length of time the peel solution was left on the skin, and the neutralizer if used. The client's response to the peel and post-care instructions along with the aesthetician's signature and date are also charted.

Safety and Sanitation: The solution for each treatment should be dispensed into a plastic medicine cup or used from the single-use vial. Excess peel solution should not be saved. Gauze sponges should be disposed of in a Ziploc bag and then trashed to eliminate fumes or harsh odors from the peel solution, which could interfere with clients and staff.

About Mary Nielsen

A technician, educator, mentor and business owner, Mary Nielsen has been at the forefront of the developments in medical esthetics since its infancy in the early 1990s. A nurse by training and experience, Mary was drawn into advanced medical esthetics with the advent of laser technologies and their use while working for a plastic surgeon. She went on to found her own successful skin and laser clinic. She is currently Vice Chair and Industry Expert on the Oregon Board of Certified Advanced Estheticians. She is the author of the advanced aesthetic textbook, A Compendium for Advanced Aesthetics, a Guide for the Master Esthetician, four books on medical spa policies and procedures, and safety policy and procedures as well as several articles on specific treatments in Skin Inc and Day Spa magazine. She is a contributor to Milady Standard Esthetics: Fundamentals, Edition 12 and writes regularly for Milady Pro.

She is the Executive Director of Spectrum Advanced Aesthetics, founder of Cascade Aesthetic Alliance, Educational Catalyst for Skintelligent Resources, and owner of Indie Aesthetics.

Contact Mary Today!

Email: mary@spectrumlasertraining.com

Chapter 4

Sensitive Skin – Understanding and Treating this Delicate Skin Type

Authored by Michele Corley

I have sensitive skin, tending towards reactive. I have put a lot of effort into finding the causes of sensitive skin, what aggravates sensitive skin, and how to address the challenges that come with this delicate skin type.

It was embarrassing for me to have such blotchy, red skin that flushed so easily. Those whom I suffer with know how it can affect self-confidence and self-esteem. The desire to better understand what was happening with my skin and how to help myself and people like me was a major factor in my decision to become an esthetician.

Throughout life, I have also been frustrated with skincare products designed for sensitive skin that still made my face itch, burn, and, on occasion, become fire-engine red – clearly this was a major influence when I started my own skincare company. My company's mission is to build confidence and self-esteem in people by creating, developing, and producing effective skincare products.

I believe that with the help of a well-educated esthetician, products that really work, and clients who are willing to be diligent with a proper home care regimen, better skin for all is possible.

I am very happy to share what I have learned about what estheticians can do to have clients confidently walking out the door with their best faces forward.

My goal in this chapter is to review the Sensitive Skin Type and Sensitized Skin Condition, the underlying characteristics of

Sensitive Skin, and my recommended Treatment Protocol for this delicate skin type.

The SENSITIVE SKIN TYPE and SENSITIZED SKIN CONDITION

Let's explore The Sensitive Skin Type and The Sensitized Skin Condition to make sure we understand them and their differences.

Sensitive Skin is a skin type that affects at least 50% of the U.S. population. Sensitive Skin has high reactivity and low tolerance of most irritants and stimuli from both internal and external sources.

Sensitive Skin is not caused by contact or reaction with any specific ingredient or material. Rather, it is an established state of the skin's inherent structure, nerve sensations, and inflammatory response. Sensitive Skin is most often linked to one or more of the following characteristics: an impaired barrier, higher neuro-sensory response, and/or chronic inflammation (frequently caused by heightened immune response).

Reactive Skin is a term for Hyper-Sensitive Skin. I consider it a subtype of Sensitive Skin. Everything that applies to Sensitive Skin applies to Reactive Skin, only more so. Reactive skin is the most volatile form of Sensitive Skin and should be handled with great care.

Sensitized Skin is a skin condition resulting from something we did to the skin as opposed to the inherent characteristics of the skin. Sensitized Skin comes about when we irritate the skin; perhaps we get sunburned or overdo it with aggressive peels.

It is important to distinguish between Sensitive Skin and Sensitized Skin. Sensitized Skin will resolve itself once the irritants are removed and the skin is given the proper care needed to repair the skin's barrier.

Now that we can distinguish between Sensitive Skin, Reactive Skin, and the Sensitized Skin condition, let's go a little deeper into the characteristics of sensitive skin.

Characteristics of Sensitive Skin

Sensitive Skin is generally characterized by thinner skin (most common in those of Northern European ancestry), which naturally has smaller sebaceous glands and therefore, predisposes one to dryer skin. Due to this common characteristic of Sensitive Skin, the skin is prone to having an impaired barrier function.

Sensitive Skin tends to have more nerves present in the stratum corneum so by its very nature it is more sensitive to stimuli than skin with a normal amount of nerves in the stratum corneum.

People with sensitive skin are also likely to have a heightened immune response which when combined with an impaired barrier and/or heightened neuro response can lead to inflammatory skin conditions such as rosacea, eczema (atopic dermatitis), and psoriasis.

Now that we understand Sensitive, Reactive, and Sensitized Skin and some of the fundamental characteristics of Sensitive Skin, let's look at how to effectively treat the Sensitive Skin Type and the Sensitized Skin condition.

Treating the Sensitive Skin Type and the Sensitized Skin Condition requires the elimination of as many irritants and triggers as possible.

Environmental, or "Choice" irritants as I call them, can include excessive sun exposure, extreme heat, extreme cold, allergens, junk food, smoking, harsh laundry detergents, and too many alcoholic beverages. Chronic stress is also a factor but, in my experience, we don't choose this level of stress, even though it sometimes chooses us.

As for skin care protocols and treatments, I recommend avoiding microdermabrasion, aggressive peels, scrubs, and any treatments or products that will severely compromise the skin's barrier.

The following is a brief list of product ingredients to avoid: Artificial Fragrance, Artificial Colorants, Essential Oils, Sodium Lauryl Sulfate, Sodium Laureth Sulfate, Alcohol, Alpha Hydroxy

Acids (with a PH below 4.5) or Beta Hydroxy Acids (with a PH below 4.5).

Let me say that I love essential oils, AHA's, and BHA's. I think microdermabrasion, peels, and scrubs are fabulous when used for the correct skin type and skin condition. However, as previously stated, I don't think any of these treatments or ingredients are appropriate for sensitive skin.

Caring for Sensitive Skin in the treatment room

We are going to address two states of sensitive skin in the following treatment. One is sensitive skin that is enraged, extremely red, hot to the touch, and very barrier compromised. The other is sensitive skin not in an extremely stressed state.

The most effective treatment protocols that our professional customer base use on clients and that we recommend at Michele Corley Clinical Skin Care are based on our Calm, Nourish, Repair and Protect Methodology. This methodology is specifically designed as a foundation for our facial protocols for barrier-impaired, sensitive, sensitized, inflamed, irritated, reactive, rosacea-prone, and eczema-prone skin.

The methodology and protocol variants focus on calming and comforting, nourishing and feeding, and repairing and fortifying sensitive or sensitized skin. We've developed products that utilize nutritious plant oils, vitamins, mineral rich clays, gentle botanicals, and protective zinc oxide to meet our standards for calming, nourishing, repairing, and ultimately, protecting the skin.

Calm, Nourish, Repair and Protect Methodology and Protocol

The following protocol utilizes Michele Corley Clinical Skin Care Products. Even if you do not have our products, you can experience good results by avoiding the aforementioned irritating ingredients and sticking to products with ingredient decks similar to ours.

Prepare the skin for treatment:

Step 1: Cleanse to remove makeup. Apply Calming Cleansing Oil & Makeup Remover to skin. Perform a cleansing massage, adding water as needed. Gently remove the cleanser (using the press and pickup method) with a lukewarm microfiber towel.

Calm, Nourish, and Repair:

Step 2: Cleanse. Apply by layering Calm, Nourish & Repair Oil & Gentle Cleansing Milk to the face, neck, and décolleté. Perform a hydrating cleansing and relaxing massage for 10 to 15 minutes, add product as necessary to maintain slip. Gently remove cleanser (using the press and pickup method) with a lukewarm microfiber towel.

Calm and Prepare for more Nourish:

Step 3: Gentle Exfoliation (SKIP STEP if skin is in an extremely irritated state). Mix Ultimate Performance Exfoliating Powder with Gentle Cleansing Milk, mix to achieve the consistency of pancake batter. Apply mask with a fan brush to the face, neck, and décolleté. Allow the client to steam 5 to 10 minutes (depending on the client's skin condition). The steamer should be approximately three feet away so that the client receives the moisture from the steam, not the heat. Remove the enzyme (using the press and pickup method) with a lukewarm microfiber towel.

Continue to Calm, Nourish, and Repair:

Step 4: Pressure Point Massage. Apply Calm, Nourish & Repair Oil to the face, neck, and décolleté and press into skin, then perform a pressure point massage for approximately 10 minutes.

Nourish, Nourish, Nourish:

Step 5: Mask. (SKIP STEP if skin is in an extremely irritated state). Mix Vitamin C Powder with Gelloid Mask. Serum may foam a bit. Apply Vitamin C Powder/Gelloid Mask mixture to the face, neck, and décolleté with a fan brush. Do not remove.

More Calm, More Nourish, and More Repair:

Step 6: Mask. Apply Calm & Hydrate Cream Mask to the face, neck, and décolleté with a fan brush. Allow mask to sit for 10 to 15 minutes. Remove mask (using the press and pickup method) with a lukewarm microfiber towel.

Step 7: Eye Care. Apply a thin layer of Age Defying Eye Cream to the orbital area of the eye.

Step 8: Serum. Apply a thin layer of Calm, Nourish & Repair Oil to the face, neck, and décolleté.

Nourish and Repair:

Step 9: Serum. (SKIP STEP if skin is in an extremely irritated state). Apply a thin layer of Vitamin C Serum Plus and/or Hyaluronic Plumping Serum to the face, neck, and décolleté.

Calm, Nourish, and Repair Some More:

Step 10: Moisturizer. Apply Calming Moisture Cream.

Calm, Nourish, Repair, and Protect:

Step 11: SPF. Apply Moisturizing SPF 30 to the face, neck, and décolleté.

Nourish and Repair your Lips:

Step 12: Lip Care. Apply Plump & Renew Lip Balm to lip area.

Thank you to all the amazing Esthetician's reading this book. I applaud your continuous effort to advance your knowledge of skin and how to best treat it. Thank you for dedicating yourselves to helping all of us walk confidently out the door.

– Michele Corley

About Michele Corley

Michele Corley is the Founder and President of Michele Corley Clinical Skin Care, a nationally distributed professional-use only skin care line based in Napa, California. Michele is a licensed Esthetician who graduated from Georgia Southern University with a bachelor's degree in business, and completed Advanced Cosmetic Chemistry at UCLA. Prior to founding and launching Michele Corley Clinical Skin Care, she earned multiple sales awards while working for a leading skincare contract manufacturer and ranked as a top sales and marketing professional.

Michele's vision is that everyone walks confidently out the door. Her mission is simple: provide efficacious products and back them up with exceptional customer service. Every Michele Corley Clinical Skin Care product is crafted with care and consideration for the health and well-being of the skin.

Michele believes in treating her clients' success as important as her own, and values everyone she has the pleasure to work with.

Info@MicheleCorley.com
707-637-4996

Chapter 5

Rezenerate NanoFacial: Obstacles, Innovation, and the Best. Facial. Ever.

Authored by Ryan Rabah

"Don't be afraid to give up the good to go for the great." –

John D. Rockefeller

The Rezenerate NanoFacial story is one of overcoming obstacles, innovating technology, and turning the "good" into the best.

In business, there are few skills that are more important than being adept at overcoming obstacles. The esthetics industry is no exception. Skin care professionals must constantly cultivate that talent: handling client demands, dealing with business operating costs, balancing personal/family time...navigating the sheer number of seemingly simple, everyday obstacles can be overwhelming. And skin care companies don't make things easier. With each claiming its product is vastly better than another, it is difficult to determine what is a good product and what is simply good marketing.

Amid this environment the Rezenerate NanoFacial Team saw an opportunity to do something innovative. The team was formed with the simple intent of helping skin care professionals overcome obstacles, but their goal was a lofty one: *Create the Best. Facial. Ever.*

REZENERATE NANOFACIAL'S MISSION

In 2013, the Rezenerate NanoFacial Team observed that product ingredient science had evolved more dramatically over the last decade than in previous years. There was an emergence of products that could heal, nourish, and improve the skin's appearance like never before. However, as is often the case, there was an obstacle. Due to our skin's waterproof barrier, these products were not achieving maximum results.

There had been no device science evolution equivalent to that of ingredient science improvements, and this became the cornerstone of the Rezenerate NanoFacial Team's mission. What if it was possible to develop a system that dramatically increased product efficacy? What if new technology could create a cosmetic facial that garnered next-level results with no negatives? What if there was an innovative modality that worked with all products and devices that skin care professionals were already utilizing? If there was a system that took an esthetician's current favorite (or best) facial and made it even better, wouldn't that become his or her "best facial ever?" This eureka moment determined the "what," but the team still needed the "how." The key to answering that question was clear...Nanotechnology.

WHAT IS NANOTECHNOLOGY?

In 1986, K. Eric Drexler wrote "Engines of Creation" and introduced the term nanotechnology to the world. Though nanotechnology has become somewhat ubiquitous in recent years, there is still confusion on its definition. In simplest terms, it means something extremely small. In scientific terms, nanotechnology is defined as "science, engineering, and technology conducted at 1 to 100 nanometers on the nanoscale."

To better understand the amazing world of nanotechnology, it is best to get an idea of the units of measure involved. A centimeter is one-hundredth of a meter, a millimeter is one-thousandth of a meter, and a micrometer is one-millionth of a meter, but these are still huge compared to the nanoscale. A nanometer (nm) is one-billionth of a meter.

So, what does this all mean? Right now, it means that scientists are experimenting with substances at the nanoscale to learn about their properties and how we can take advantage of them in various applications. Scientists and engineers are having great success making materials at the nanoscale to take advantage of enhanced properties such as higher strength, lighter weight, and improved performance.

Rezenerate NanoFacial decided to utilize that technology in the world of esthetics.

REZENERATE NANOFACIAL BENEFITS

The Rezenerate NanoFacial is a new skin care modality that delivers the results of more invasive systems without the negatives. Its NanoFacial Modality safely conditions in the stratum corneum. The Rezenerate WandPro is a handheld device that uses individual, single-use only tips, called Rezenerate NanoFacial Chips (or Tips), to perform cosmetic facials. Rezenerate's pain free, non-invasive facial means no numbing cream is required and it's safe to use on lips and sensitive areas, and even up to the lash line. Rezenerate NanoFacial's resounding success is centered around a 3-Phased system of '**Stratum Disruption**.'

Phase 1 - Vibratory Facial Massage

This is the initial phase of the Rezenerate NanoFacial. The WandPro motor's vibrations lead to increased blood circulation, which stimulates skin and encourages natural oxygenation, producing a complexion with a healthy and natural glow. Often, tense facial expressions mean more wrinkles, so Rezenerate's vibratory NanoFacial massage is beneficial for tension relief and provides an instant plumping and reduction of fine lines.

Phase 2 - Product Infusion

No two individuals have the same skin nutrient needs. Rezenerate NanoFacial allows you to customize a facial solution for your client using the products you already know and love. The middle phase of the NanoFacial is best explained through an acronym Rezenerate coined: **N.A.N.O. (Non-Ablative Nutrient Optimization)**.

The Rezenerate NanoFacial optimizes skin health by delivering the nutrients in the products you already use and love without any discomfort or net negative. This is the "Nutrient Optimization" component.

Think about this: Would a doctor recommend only taking 10% percent of your daily vitamin? Of course not! And yet average industry absorption rates for products when using other modalities typically fall between 2% to 10%. During the Rezenerate NanoFacial, a clients' skin becomes a "sponge" and serum/products are absorbed better than ever before. A Rezenerate NanoFacial can increase absorption to upwards of 40% to 50%, thereby optimizing the nutrient benefits of a skin care professional's chosen products.

The "Non-Ablative" component is self-explanatory. The Rezenerate NanoFacial does all of this without pain or discomfort. During the NanoFacial more than a million invisible "Rezenerate Nanochannels" are created in the stratum corneum. Rezenerate minimizes inflammation and the body's immune response by using a gentle approach to skin nutrition.

Phase 3 - Accelerated Exfoliation

This final phase of the Rezenerate NanoFacial typically occurs over 2-4 days post facial.

The stratum corneum is comprised of layers of keratin-rich corneocyte cells (keratinocytes). Keratinocytes shed naturally in the process called desquamation. As we age, the glue-like intercellular cement holding the cells together becomes denser, causing a build-up in the layers of cells.

As cell desquamation becomes more difficult, skin appears duller, thicker, and less toned. Rezenerate's gentle 'Stratum Disruption' process accelerates and enhances natural desquamation.

The results have not gone unnoticed.

Per industry leader Shelley Hancock, "The Rezenerate [NanoFacial] has exceeded my expectations! The new cutting edge Rezenerate [NanoFacial] treatment is the ultimate in anti-aging...your skin is more hydrated...pigmentation lightening, toning, and an overall youthful glow to your skin."

While clients walk out of a Rezenerate NanoFacial feeling and looking amazing, the true benefits have just begun. Rezenerate acts as a catalyst, assisting and enhancing the products, serums, and other modalities you already use that address your clients' various skin issues. It does this by employing its two core concepts: Product Neutrality and Modality Neutrality.

REZENERATE NANOFACIAL'S CORE CONCEPTS

Core Concept 1 - Product Neutrality

Rezenerate NanoFacial does not sell its own product line nor does it promote any specific product line. Rezenerate Leadership felt that would be disingenuous because the system works well with any high-level product line. Rezenerate believes estheticians and other skin care professionals are the experts in determining which specific products to use on each client.

"Rezenerate understands there is no one-size-fits-all skin care solution and foregoes potential product line sales for professional integrity.   Those are the types of companies I like to partner with...ones that don't strictly push a "sales" agenda, but rather put estheticians first.   That's a big part of Rezenerate's success," says Sheri Flasch, Esthetics Influencer and founder of the Esthetician Connection (www.estheticianconnection.com).

In fact, Rezenerate NanoFacial achieves its amazing results due to the array of incredible skin care lines, some of which you may already work with.   This is part of their Product Neutrality core concept.   By collaborating with the top skin care lines on the market today, Rezenerate NanoFacial is proud to be at the helm of unprecedented results-oriented facials.

Product Neutrality gives skin care professionals options to improve their clients' issues.   Whichever products are used, Rezenerate NanoFacial will dramatically increase its effectiveness. The Rezenerate NanoFacial makes professional products better, including peptides, lactics, glycolics, hyaluronics, stem cells, antioxidants, mandelics, and more.   Estheticians can customize treatments like never before, which leads to better outcomes.

Core Concept 2 - Modality Neutrality

Many professionals ask what existing modality the Rezenerate NanoFacial is displacing, but that question is looking through the lens of an outdated paradigm. Rezenerate does not want to replace anything on the market, instead, it can be used in conjunction or "stacked" with all other modalities. As a professional, you can pair the Rezenerate NanoFacial with microdermabrasion, LED, dermaplane, peels, and high frequency to name only a few.

Rezenerate NanoFacial acts as a catalyst, allowing you to increase your customer base. It is perfect for clients who typically want the results of an aggressive facial, but with none of the negatives.

A NEW OBSTACLE EMERGES: IMITATORS

Another obstacle Rezenerate NanoFacial had to overcome was the birth of imitators. The adage of imitation being the sincerest form of flattery has proven unequivocally untrue. "Our legal department has had to file suit or send cease-and-desist letters to a number of unethical companies trying to trade off our name or promote copycat, inferior products. It's like a game of Whack-a-Mole," said Jaylene Cosme, Office Manager at Rezenerate NanoFacial in Charlotte, NC.

With innovation, the market becomes filled with inferior products (typically created overseas). And as false information spreads, Rezenerate always strives to share facts to keep the record straight.

Many companies have begun using the term "nano" as a marketing buzz word, but they do not utilize actual nanotechnology science in their products, nor do they understand nanotechnology concepts when asked. As one might expect, they do not offer any guarantee that they use verified nanotechnology (like the Nanotechnology Certificate that comes with the Rezenerate NanoFacial system).

Further, because both are similar looking handheld devices, a common misconception imitators exploit is that the Rezenerate NanoFacial WandPro is similar to microneedling devices. It is important to note the Rezenerate NanoFacial is NOT any form of microneedling but is its own modality. As such, a NanoFacial cannot be performed with a repurposed microneedling device as some companies claim. Adjustable devices are developed for needles, which allow for a large margin of error without changing the overall result as they are trying to create a wound cascade. The Rezenerate NanoFacial WandPro device does not adjust and is made specifically for the Rezenerate NanoFacial Tips.

Due to companies that unethically claim to sell devices that perform both microneedling and NanoFacials, and because there are so many esthetic devices on the market, education was needed on the regulatory and policy-making levels. For example, an inspector visited and fined a Rezenerate Authorized Provider (RAP) in California after mistaking the Rezenerate WandPro for a microneedling device. The RAP reached out to Wendy Jacobs, an esthetician advocate and founder of the California Aesthetic Alliance, to investigate for Rezenerate NanoFacial users in California.

According to Wendy, she "presented the Rezenerate

NanoFacial to members of the California Board of Barbering and Cosmetology to explain that it is actual nanotechnology, no other tips are made for Rezenerate Wands, and depth cannot be changed on the device. The result? The fine was reversed and Rezenerate NanoFacial has been found to be well within the scope of practice for California licensed estheticians."

While the imitation adage fell short, there is one that always holds true: you get what you pay for. If it doesn't say Rezenerate NanoFacial, then it simply isn't.

THE REZENERATE NANOFACIAL FUTURE

Rezenerate NanoFacial is proud to be a company that innovates and overcomes obstacles. The best way to determine what happens in the future is to create the future yourself. That is what Rezenerate NanoFacial has done and that is what they are inviting skin care professionals all over the country to do.

The advent of nanotechnology applications will be the world's next industrial revolution, and Rezenerate NanoFacial is excited to be part of that bright future by bringing the benefits of verified

nanotechnology to the world of esthetics. Those deciding to join

the 'Rezenerate Revolution' by adding the NanoFacial to their list

of services place themselves on the forefront of a new disruptive

industry technology and will start to turn the "good" into the Best.

(Facial. Ever.).

About Ryan Rabah

Ryan is the President and Co-founder of Rezenerate. Born in Houston, TX and raised in Queens, NY, Ryan has happily settled in Charlotte, NC. In addition to heading the team at Rezenerate NanoFacial, Ryan is a licensed attorney, focusing on Business, Real Estate, and Esthetics Law and is proud to be the inaugural Member of the Esthetician Connection Advisory Board (www.estheticianconnection.com).

When not hard at work supporting estheticians, filing documents, and promoting the Best.Facial.Ever., Ryan can be found writing profusely, reading incessantly, and spending as much time as time possible with his best friend and daughter Jade Katherine.

www.rezenerate.com
info@rezenerate.com
754.800.4ZEN

Chapter 6

Personalized Color Theory

Authored by Jaclyn Peresetsky

I began my career as a professionally trained artist. Then, I decided I was in love with the beauty and complexity of the face, so I focused on portrait artistry. During every commissioned portrait, I was always fascinated by the beauty of skin color and how all of us are so uniquely created from our genetics.

Have you ever thought about your own personal coloring or your client's?

This subject is complicated and many of us don't learn about the complex relationship between color and the human being. When we consider factors that affect our skin, we learn about intrinsic and extrinsic factors. Color's effect on the human being can be considered in the same way. People have internal complexities in the natural coloring of eyes, skin, and hair, which are dictated by genetics. Furthermore, that color has psychological, emotional, and physiological effects.

Estheticians make decisions every day that are affected by the complexity of skin tone. Every person we work on has unique coloring. However, we all have the same basic ingredients: melanin (pigment of the skin varying from brown, blue-brown, red-brown, and green-brown), hemoglobin (blood varying from blue-red to reddish pink), and carotene (the yellow pigmentation of the skin varying from yellow to yellow-orange). What makes an individual's skin color unique is the concentration of the melanin in relation to the slight variances of hemoglobin and carotene.

Melanin is the main factor influencing skin color. While people of different ethnicities have similar numbers of melanocytes, the variation of skin tone is heavily influenced by the amount of pigment produced by the melanocyte. For example, large amounts of melanin produce black skin and low producing melanocytes produce pale yellow skin.

Carotenoids are brightly colored substances found in egg yolks and vegetables such as carrots, chard, peppers, and others. Carotene is yellowy-orange and is a powerful antioxidant that helps protect skin cells from oxidative damage. In the body, it is transformed into vitamin A, which is essential for vision and good skin health. Have you heard of a baby eating too much carrot baby food and getting orange cheeks? Well, this can happen because of the carotene rich carrots.

Hemoglobin is a molecule in the blood that carries oxygen, lending the skin a reddish pink color. Where the hemoglobin is not picking up enough oxygen from the lungs and carrying it around the body, the skin can appear blue, sallow, or grey. Therefore, circulatory and respiratory health reflects visually through skin cells. Many chronic lung conditions like emphysema can make the skin look blue or grey.

So, now that we have gone over the science of skin tone, let's cover what dictates unique blends of melanin, hemoglobin, and carotene for everyone. I am sure you have heard how important your genes are in determining skin tone. An individual's skin and hair color are clues to his or her ancestry and heritage. Skin and hair color is primarily determined by the genes we inherit from our parents. In fact, if your parents experienced premature greying (in their 20's or 30's), then it is likely your hair will grey sooner rather than later. How your skin reacts to UV exposure is also dictated by your genetics. When I see clients for skin evaluations, I always ask how each of their parents react to prolonged sun exposure. Then, I can usually tell which parent their skin relates to more. I can also be more aware of skin cancer history, sunburn history, and any unique skin reactions. It's important to know as much as possible about your client's ancestry. We are lucky with today's technology that with a simple spit test, one can find out all the details about his or her heritage. The natural amount of melanin in an individual's skin can be a contraindication for certain chemical peels or laser procedures. A specific tone to be wary of is olive undertones; they have what I call "sneaky melanin". Determining a client's skin tone and his or her heritage is crucial to understanding how to best treat his or her skin. So, why wouldn't identifying undertone be important in understanding makeup colors to best compliment your client's complexion and features?

As estheticians and makeup artists, we sift through hundreds of makeup colors to find the right shades for our clients. Have you ever thought you chose the right makeup base, but at the end of the makeup application you realize everything seems off? You run through your calculated steps and look at your makeup color choices so elegantly displayed in front of the client to see where the misstep was. Little do most beauty professionals realize, the initial foundation choice did not have the correct undertone to harmonize with the clients' skin. Almost every step thereafter was incorrect. Some makeup pros pretend that undertone does not matter and believe every person can wear yellow, pink, beige, and olive tones. Other makeup pros love the artistry through the creative application of makeup but forgo the due diligence to check undertone. Over the last decade, I have focused on studying undertone and the effects makeup color or hair color choices have on the skin. There are some specific identifiers and tests artists can use to categorize colors, which help identify the colors that harmonize with specific skin tones.

First, you need to identify if the client is warm, cool, warm neutral, or cool neutral. This may sound confusing, but there are tried-and-true quick tests to help. One test is to have your client apply orange lipstick (warm shade), purple lipstick (cool shade), coral lipstick (neutral warm shade), and pink lipstick (neutral cool shade). Take a picture of the client in each lipstick color with a smart phone. Then, slide the pictures back and forth until you choose which shade looks the best. Another way to identify this color characteristic is to use a set of shades of white drapes. First, drape an ivory scarf (warm shade), pure white scarf (cool shade), off-white scarf (neutral warm shade), and winter white/grey white scarf (neutral cool shade) over the client. Again, take pictures of each shade. Then, slide the pictures back and forth to decide. The best picture should be obvious. The right shade of white will make clients look younger and brighter, and their complexions will look smoother. Keep in mind, lighting is crucial so you must have full spectrum lighting or be near a window to be the most accurate. You need to know if a client is warm, cool, warm neutral, or cool neutral because this gives you a better idea of the color palette you should choose from for makeup, hair, and clothing. For example, if a client is warm, any makeup in the warm family will look great. In fact, the warm makeup colors will harmonize with her skin and make it look like she has on very little makeup, naturally enhancing her features.

Next, you should identify what color, or hue, is most dominant in the client's skin. Every skin tone has a combination of yellow (carotene), brown (melanin that can be greenish brown-olive, greyish brown-beige, or ochre brown), and red (hemoglobin). One color is usually dominant, which gives you his or her undertone. The easiest way to determine this is by swiping foundation shades that are dominant in these undertones along the jawline and identifying which one blends in effortlessly. Keep in mind, the value (the lightness or darkness of a shade) can vary if a client has a tan, but the undertone of the skin always holds true. For example, I am typically a medium light value. When I use pigment lighteners

71

or bleaching creams in my skincare regiment, my skin may lighten. After sun exposure, my skin will be slightly darker. These are important things to keep in mind when clients are concerned about a foundation shade being too dark or too light. I always recommend they buy two foundations with their skincare goals in mind. For example, if they are doing a lot of chemical peels or using aggressive skincare products that focus on lightening sun spots, they may want to choose a shade that matches the current value of their skin and an additional shade that is lighter if their skin changes. They can use either shade or mix them. If a client works outside or has plans to go on a sunny vacation, she may buy a shade that matches her current tone and a darker shade to mix and match. Referring back to undertone biology, it is genetic and does not change unless from an illness such as a liver condition (increasing yellow/green), hypertension (increasing red), or emphysema (increasing grey), etc. I happen to have a lot of yellow in my skin which makes me truly warm, so I always need a golden foundation shade. In fact, when I have tried other shades, my skin tone looks ashy, sick, or tired. Therefore, golden shades are the best for my skin tone. I like to place foundation shades into 4 categories: yellow, peach, beige, and olive. The key is to swipe the right value in each of the 4 undertone categories side by side along the jawline of your client. Whichever shade disappears in their skin is the winner. Once again, lighting is vital and you must have full spectrum lighting or natural light for accuracy. Once this is complete, you know the undertone of the client's skin and you can confidently choose the foundation that will only enhance the skin's natural beauty. Consequently, remaining makeup choices will also look beautiful. I recommend explaining this process to clients so they understand how you chose the right shade. Once you educate them about their undertone, they will be impressed by your due diligence and will trust you in future makeup selections.

Finally, if you want to make exact color choices or recommendations for your client's undertone, you may want to consider adding a color analysis service to your spa/salon menu. This additional service can set you apart as a color expert and allow you to explore other services or products to recommend. As stated earlier, color analysis can be done through draping a client in different fabrics or simultaneously comparing one color against another. Full spectrum lighting or natural light are imperative for proper color analysis. You may want to invest in this extensive service. There are many different systems that you can consider. For example, the traditional color analysis system that started with the book Color Me Beautiful focuses on the four-season palettes. More extensive and detailed color analysis systems focus on twelve to sixteen palettes. These more extensive systems focus on secondary color characteristics such as light, dark, bright, soft, delicate, or bold. At the end of color analysis services, your clients should get a swatch booklet of their best colors so they can easily choose the best makeup, nail, or clothing colors. This would make it easy for you to make the right color choices for spa/salon services.

Overall, clients want to look younger, brighter and more refreshed. Color is a simple way to do this while also providing immediate gratification. Understanding clients' undertones is essential in choosing suitable colors that allow their best attributes to shine. If you have never considered an identification technique to determine your client's undertone, then you are truly missing out on elevating your professionalism and brand. Save yourself time, money, and frustration by becoming a beauty expert who knows how to harmonize color with a client's undertone. Honing this skill must be a priority, thereby, making you the leading expert in your field!

About Jaclyn Peresetsky

Jaclyn Peresetsky is not only the owner of Skin Perfect Spas in Ohio and Florida, but she is also a noted

color expert, makeup artist, master esthetician, permanent makeup instructor, author, and speaker. Her multiple books, cosmetic and skin care lines, and training courses allow other beauty pros to learn and add more services that combine art and science to become leading beauty experts. Her passion for education led her to create a school for Advanced Esthetics and Color, opening in January of 2019 in Columbus, OH

Contact Info:

Jaclyn Peresetsky

Owner of Skin Perfect Spas & Colore Me Perfect Cosmetics

www.skinperfectclinic.com

www.coloremeperfect.com

Office: 239-262-5110
jaclyn@skinperfectclinic.com

Chapter 7

Educating the Future, a Perspective From an Aesthetics School Owner

Authored by Felicia Tyler

At the age of 24, I opened my first day spa in Naperville, IL in 1999. It was an exciting time. I was young, passionate, and eager to show the world what I could do. Always an entrepreneur at heart, I aimed to separate myself from the competition and try something different. There were many local day spas in the area and my background at that time was in midwifery; I knew I could create my own niche. My husband (fiancé at the time) and I had gone to college in south Florida and during the midwifery program, I had completed an externship in Colombia and delivered well over 200 babies throughout my career. After graduation, I managed a birthing center in Hollywood, Florida until deciding to move back to Illinois for my husband's work. Unfortunately, Illinois home birth laws did not allow me to continue to work as I had hoped but it did present another opportunity. I had a career decision to make and felt that massage therapy was a natural transition because I could specialize in pregnancy and induction massages. My day spa began almost immediately after graduation from massage therapy school and it was popular with the local community from day one. I was the go-to person for everyone's massage and pregnancy care but always lacked a qualified skin care staff. Because of the vision I had for the business, I knew something had to change. So, in 2001, I enrolled in aesthetics school.

While I was in aesthetics school, I received a basic skin care education and I quickly realized why my skin care staff was lacking the proper skill set and knowledge. It also raised questions about my local competitors and why they were all offering basic skin care services as well. Were they just sticking to a tried and true service menu that worked or was it that all the aestheticians coming out of school were trained in just the basics? All I knew for sure was that I wanted to offer something better. The goal was to be the go-to person not just for massage and pregnancy care, but for skin care. I wanted to accomplish this by understanding ingredients, formulations, advanced protocols, industry trends, and even nutrition. I knew there had to be more advanced techniques than using just a lactic acid peel. Upon graduation from aesthetics school, I began to split my time between running my day spa and taking every advanced skin care continuing education class that I could find.

Thankfully, my clients responded positively to my continued skin care education. They knew I was serious about education and training and felt that I had a talent for skin care. Clients wanted me to help them find their youthful glow again, help their teenagers with acne and scarring, or simply recommend an eye cream that their husbands could use. During sessions, clients would ask me about skin care and how it relates to nutrition. Another popular topic would be peel and microdermabrasion combination treatments and how they related to minimizing pores and fine lines. Also, everyone wanted to know what product was in my purse that I couldn't live without. These conversations would have been great topics for a blog but unfortunately, there were no social media back then. Today's information highway makes everyone so much more informed and technical knowledge makes every aesthetician that much better.

Back then, clients fell in love with my simple crystal microdermabrasion machine or basic glycolic and lactic acid peels. At the time, none of my local competitors were offering any of these services. We were getting busier and busier and needed to hire more qualified help. I was interviewing everyone that would answer my help-wanted ads and quickly realized that everyone had just a basic skin care education. Most applicants had never performed a chemical peel let alone seen a microdermabrasion machine. I clearly remember having one crystal microdermabrasion machine that would get clogged every couple of weeks. It was embarrassing having to cancel clients for a few days until I could get the machine fixed. It didn't help that my skin care staff did not know how to properly use or clean the machine either. Clients were so nice and patient but they were certainly annoyed. It was great having a service menu item that everyone always booked, if only it could stop clogging. Looking back now, I cringe at these times before diamond tip machines were available.

The business was growing but I was spending most my time training new staff. It was time consuming, but it was very rewarding to see others perform above their own expectations with just a little bit of guidance. It was during this time that my husband and I started talking about the future and the direction we wanted the business to go. Always with the entrepreneur mindset, we started talking about the possibility of opening our own school. The initial objective was to offer students an education based on the proper technical training that was expected of them in the real world. Our hope was that we would have a successful school and respected brand; we were right. Together, my husband and I decided to dedicate the next year of our lives into understanding where the line existed between educational curriculum and the real-world expectation for a skin care school graduate.

Now, the journey began. We started by sending out questionnaires and surveys to local day spas asking for their feedback on whether their aestheticians had the skill set required upon being hired. We talked with our own clients to get a better understanding of their customer service needs. My husband and I also began traveling to see what skin care practices were popular in different parts of the country. We attended lots of industry events and concluded the journey by visiting local skin care programs. We compared the type of skin care education schools were offering at the time vs. the expectations of graduates in the real world. It was a very exciting time and we gained real perspective on how to develop a technically advanced aesthetics program for our new school.

In 2005, we decided to sell the day spa and focus full-time on opening a school. In 2006, we opened the doors of our first school, "Universal Spa Training Academy", located in Downers Grove, IL. The curriculum was created based upon the requirements of aestheticians in the real world.

Today, we have graduated over one thousand students and offer the strongest aesthetics program in Illinois. The school has wonderful partnerships with the area's doctors, mentorship programs, externships, cosmetic companies, permanent makeup providers, and employers. We are a frequent destination for continuing education hours and have students traveling across state lines to attend the program. Our aesthetics program includes all technical areas that give graduates an advantage over their competition. Students learn about enzymes, AHA's, BHA's, TCA's, Jessner's, microcurrent, individual lash extensions, DermaDisc, ultrasound, ultrasonic skin scrubber, laser hair removal, dermaplaning, micro-needling, oncology treatments, cosmetic lasers, LED treatments, IPL's and more.

Like the feeling I had training staff in my day spa, my husband and I both get tremendous satisfaction watching the graduates go on to be successful on their own. We were recently speaking with a very well-known and respected plastic surgeon in Chicago. He informed us that one of our past graduates is now running his entire aesthetics department. He was impressed with her skill set and overall knowledge, which made us feel great because she is such a fantastic person.

When I graduated from aesthetics' school, the basic career path was to work independently, work in a spa, salon or hotel, or teach. All are great career tracks, but now graduates have endless choices. They are successful in finding work as medical aestheticians, laser technicians, product line representatives, lash experts, permanent make-up artists, business owners, make-up artists, expert bloggers, consultants, trainers for product lines and medical spas, office managers, department heads and our personal favorite, entrepreneurs!

In 2018, we are opening our newest location, The Spa Training Academy, in Sarasota, Florida. Just like what we saw in Illinois 12 years ago, the skill set of skin care therapists in Florida is lacking and my husband and I are looking forward to elevating the education standards there as well. We hope that you enjoyed learning a bit about the technical advances of this industry as it relates to education.

About Felicia Tyler

Felicia Tyler is the co-founder of Universal Spa Training Academy and The Spa Training Academy, a chain of nationally accredited beauty and wellness schools. Felicia holds a degree in midwifery and is a licensed esthetician, instructor, and massage therapist. She lives in the Chicagoland area with 2 children, a husband, and a house full of animals. Felicia is a published author, mentor, and education advocate with over 20 years of experience.

Contact Felicia at: felicia@spatrainingacademy.com

www.spatrainingacademy.edu

Chapter 8

Manual Facial Lymphatic Drainage Massage

Authored by Michele Phelan, LE, RA, CIDESCO

Manual Facial Lymphatic Drainage massage (MFLD) has become a popular procedure for estheticians to perform during their skin care treatments. It has also been used by therapists around the world for years to help provide their clients with its multifaceted benefits. The original and perhaps, the most popular method of lymphatic drainage was invented by a Danish doctor, Emil Vodder, and his wife Estrid in 1932. It is called the "Vodder method" and is practiced worldwide. Other experts of lymphatic drainage have since added their unique spins to this therapeutic procedure, and alternative modalities to the manual method are also used today.

If implemented correctly by a knowledgeable therapist, MFLD can provide outstanding healing effects. It can be administered as a stand-alone procedure or as an addition to your skin care treatment to increase efficacy. Prior to performing this healing therapy, you should first understand the lymphatic system and the massage technique itself. It can take weeks of training and practice to become good, and years of practice to become an expert in MFLD. For this reason, if you wish to practice full-face or body lymphatic drainage it would benefit you to take a hands-on course. However, in this chapter I will teach you the basics of the lymphatic system and briefly describe the MFLD technique. I will give you a simple protocol for decreasing puffy eyes at the end of this chapter.

A Little About the Lymphatic and Circulatory Systems:

The lymphatic system is closely related to the cardiovascular (circulatory) system; the two work in conjunction with each other. The lymphatic system's main goal is to absorb, clean, and carry lymph back to the circulatory system, as well as help to provide a consistent balance of fluid in the tissue. The lymphatic system is comprised of many lymph vessels and other lymphoid tissue. Lymph fluid is mostly comprised of water, proteins, and white blood cells (lymphocytes). It is the lymphocytes that help defend the body against disease.

You can think of the lymphatic system as the detoxification system for the tissue of the body. Lymph vessels move in only one direction, toward the heart. Lymph moves quite slowly through the body and is stimulated naturally by movement and breathing. Once lymph fluid has been picked up by tiny lymph capillaries and transferred to lymph vessels, it begins its journey back to the heart through a network called the lymphatic system. A large portion of the lymphatic system is quite superficial in the tissue, but it also surrounds internal organs. The fluid is cleaned by lymphocytes, which engulf pathogens and destroy them. As lymph fluid moves back to the heart, it stops in lymph nodes along the way that contain a great amount of lymphocytes. The fluid also slows down as it moves through the lymph nodes, which ensures that bacteria, viruses, and other pathogens are removed before the lymph re-joins the circulatory system.

On the other hand, the circulatory system has two sides to its network. One side is the artery side that carries oxygen, water and nutrient enriched blood away from the heart and out to the tissues for nourishment. The other side is the vein side that brings deoxygenated blood back to the heart to gain more oxygen and nutrients. The red blood cells (erythrocytes), a type of cell that populates the circulatory system, carry oxygen and iron. As a quick reminder, medical charts show the arteries as red vessels and the veins as blue.

Lymph fluid is seepage or diffusion of the circulatory system. When this fluid is in the circulatory system it is called plasma. When it diffuses into the tissue from the circulatory system it is called interstitial fluid. Interstitial fluid protects cells, bathes cells, and helps carry nutrients in and toxins out of cells. It also helps to keep a normal balance of fluid in the tissue. Edema is a result of too much interstitial fluid in one area and can indicate inflammation or injury. Removal of protein in the tissue is essential because too much can draw water and cause swelling. When fluid eventually diffuses into lymph vessels from tissue it is called lymph. At this point, lymph fluid begins its journey back to the heart to re-join the circulatory system, and the cycle starts over.

Lymphatic fluid re-joins the circulatory system in the clavicle region. In this region, there is one duct on each side of the body that transports all the lymph back into the circulatory system. I like to think of it as the gateway from the lymphatic system to the circulatory system. The duct on the right side of the body is the lymphatic duct, and on the left side is the thoracic duct. The thoracic duct has a greater job than the lymphatic duct because it takes in most of the returning lymph, excluding the lymph from the right side of the head, face, right arm, and thoracic region. This portion is cleared by the right lymphatic duct instead. Together, these ducts are sometimes known as the "terminus". Place your fingers on both earlobes and draw a straight line down to right above your collar bone; this is the terminus region. These two points should receive a small amount of stimulation or light pumping before an MFLD. This will help clear or open channels before starting the massage technique. It is necessary to stimulate the terminus prior to lymphatic drainage so that lymph flow does not back up in the channels and cause stagnation; think of it as "opening the flood gates."

Because lymphatic drainage speeds up lymph fluid travel through the system, often twenty times faster than normal, it can accelerate healing by stimulating the immune system, ridding the system of toxins, and reducing swelling and inflammation. It is one of the best massage techniques to help treat the following conditions, providing the client does not have any known contraindications.

* Puffy, swollen eyes

* Edema after cosmetic facial surgery (once thoroughly trained)

* Inflammation after a skin extraction treatment

* Retention of fluid due to excess consumption of salt or sugar (two hygroscopic ingredients)

* Low energy level

* Color and tone of the skin

Below is a list of many contraindications (not limited to) you should make sure the client does not have before this massage:

1. **Cancer**

2. **Thyroid disease and other glandular disorders**

3. **HIV (check with the doctor)**

4. **Kidney disease**

5. **Heart disease**

6. **Congestive heart and other heart conditions**

7. **Blood clots**

8. **Asthma**

9. **Pregnancy or breast feeding**

10. **Viruses**

When we perform lymphatic drainage for the skin we are concerned with the superficial lymphatics. Unlike other types of massage, lymphatic drainage is more like a feather touch. While performing MFLD to the face there are several things to keep in mind. First, lymph mainly enters the capillary at the initial lymphatic (the beginning of a capillary). Pressure needs to be very light to avoid closing down this portion of the capillary. From one lymph vessel valve to the next is called the lymphangion. Each lymphangion has an internal stretch sensor. When the skin is stretched in the direction that you want the fluid to flow and then released, the vessels vacuum the lymph and move it efficiently through the vessel.

Touch should be so very light that you don't even feel the client's bone beneath your fingertips. A stretching and release technique is used. Fingers should neither move across the skin nor press into the skin. Movement should be slow and rhythmic. Stimulation of the terminus should always take place first and then the area closest to the terminus should be drained. As you begin to move away from the terminus, movement should still be in the direction of the terminus. This will ensure that the lymph is flowing in the correct direction. Generally, each area that you are working on should be drained at least 3 times for the greatest benefit.

Directions for mini under eye massage:

To help reduce under-eye puffiness. Note: Prior to draining the eye area, perform a light downward feather touch massage on the neck and then on the lower face (with outward/downward strokes on the face). This prepares the eye area to carry fluid down and away from region.

In the under-eye area, the lymph naturally flows laterally and slightly inferiorly. With two massage fingers on the lateral side of each under eye, stretch the *skin laterally (out) and slightly inferiorly (down), simultaneously, creating a half moon stretch, and then release*. Perform this technique five times in three areas under the eye beneath the tear trough. Start at the outer corner of the under eye then move directly beneath the mid portion of the under eye and lastly the most medial portion of the under eye. Next drain the upper eye area. Starting at the outside (tail) of the eyebrow, use your massage fingers. Slightly tug on the eyebrow skin laterally five times. Next perform this technique to the mid portion of the eyebrow and lastly to the most medial portion. At the close of this massage, perform light lateral effleurage strokes on the forehead and once again, down the face and neck lightly.

About Michele Phelan

Michele Phelan has been a licensed esthetician for over 30 years and a CIDESCO diplomat for over 15. She has had several skin care clinics and a full service spa located in San Francisco, Ca. Michele still maintains a semi-full time skin care practice. She has taught esthetics at every level including: state board, CIDESCO, and other medical and clinical curriculum. She has served as a CIDESCO examiner and helped to develop the CIDESCO curriculum at Ms. Marty's beauty college, the first college in California to have this acclaimed international program. Michele is a sought after guest speaker at esthetics symposiums around the nation. She is also a registered aromatherapist.

Michele developed and founded Concepts Institute of Advanced Esthetics. Here, she writes and teaches the core curriculum for the Clinical Esthetics course and in conjunction with Dr. Bradley Greene, MD, MBA FACS, writes and teaches part of the Para-medical esthetics course. In 2017, the duo launched their on-line para-medical esthetics course so that it would be available to estheticians nationally and globally. She has authored many articles in such publications as Dermascope, Skin Inc. Skin Deep, Les Nouvelle on topics such as medical esthetics, aromatherapy, modalities, skin care ingredients and business to name a few.

Contact Michele Today!
Concepts Institute of Advanced Esthetics
Address: 341 West Lake Center (medical/dental Bldg.) #245
Daly City (Bay Area), CA 94015
Email: conceptsmmp@gmail.com
Website: http://www.conceptsinstitute.com

Chapter 9

A Brief Overview of Skin Lightening Ingredients and How They Work

Authored by Michael Q. Pugliese, LE
Circadia by Dr. Pugliese, Inc.

As skin care professionals, we are frequently presented with clients' skin concerns relating to hyperpigmentation disorders, or the uneven distribution of visible melanin in the skin. The source of this spotty disarray can be a combination of factors, with sun exposure being universally recognized as a primary cause. Evidence of adolescent inflammatory acne may be present decades later, compounding damage from new breakouts at the onset of mid-life.

In men and women, hormonal fluctuations, smoking, and a history of excessive/aggressive treatments are known to trigger the production of melanin. The biomedical research of skin mechanisms that create melanin have allowed a discerning look into the topical agents currently in the professional skin care market, used across skin types and age ranges.

For this chapter, I will introduce the basic principles of this complex subject, then discuss several skin lightening ingredients and formulation technologies categorized by their method of action.

In studying this specific skin care concern, keep in mind that all clients seeking your help are best served by proper esthetic treatments, along with an integrated approach that considers medical history, lifestyle, client commitment, and compliant at-home care.

Melanogenesis

Human skin color comes from the outermost layer of the skin, the epidermis, where the pigment-producing cells called melanocytes are localized to produce melanin. When stimulated by an environmental or mechanical insult, melanin is produced in the skin as a protective response. This process, called melanogenesis, is enhanced by the activation of a key enzyme, tyrosinase. Tyrosinase is a glycoprotein located in the membrane of the melanosome. Two types of melanin called eumelanin and pheomelanin are synthesized within the melanosome. Eumelanin is a dark brown-black insoluble polymer, whereas pheomelanin is a light, red-yellow, Sulphur-containing soluble polymer. The production of these materials inside the melanocyte is referred to as the dark-pathway and the light-pathway, respectively. In general, melanin production in the skin can be broken down into two categories: constitutive, which is determined by genetics, and facultative, which results from an induced source.

Many other bioactive molecules are involved in the synthesis of melanin for photoprotection; this is only a brief introduction to a complex subject. Because treating uneven skin tone is an important aspect of esthetic practice, it is critical that practitioners seek out additional references, trainings, and current treatments to further their understanding of the factors causing pigmentation. As estheticians, we need to continue to explore evolving concepts and better ways to help clients achieve their goals.

Inhibition of Tyrosinase

As mentioned, tyrosinase is a glycoprotein found within the melanocyte and its inhibition is the most prominent and widely used technique available to skincare specialists for skin lightening. Most skin-lightening ingredients today fit into this category of skin lighteners. **Hydroquinone** is still considered the standard for short term results in the United States but is currently banned in most other parts of the world that regulate cosmetics. For many years, the U.S. industry has also been moving away from using hydroquinone due to its documented ability to induce reactive oxygen species and quinones, leading to oxidative damage of membrane lipids and proteins. Exogenous ochronosis in higher Fitzpatrick types is also a major concern for those using higher concentrations over long spans of time. These factors have given rise to many innovative developments among skin lighteners that are also categorized as tyrosinase inhibitors. **Alpha-arbutin** is a glycosylated form of hydroquinone, and although it is chemically very different, it is recognized as an effective and suitable alternative to HQ without potential risks. **Kojic acid**, **azelaic acid**, and **gentisic acid** have also been used for many years with little to no complications.

Vitamin C (A2A) in any stable form is recognized as an effective skin lightener, however, the unstable nature of A2A has led formulators to seek alternative options to achieve optimal results. The more stable ascorbate ester, magnesium-1-ascorbyl-2-phosphate (MAP) is lipophilic and has a greater permeation through the stratum corneum. Tetrahexyldecyl ascorbate has been clinically shown to lighten skin in as low as 1% concentration.

Botanical blends including *bearberry*, *paper mulberry*, and *licorice extracts* (due to its content of *glabradin)* have been shown to be highly effective skin lighteners because of their ability to function as tyrosinase inhibitors. More recent data has shown *Rumex Occidentalis* extract, a plant indigenous to Canada, to be even more active than licorice.

Next Generation Tyrosinase inhibitors

The demand to develop highly effective skin lighteners has led to significant technological advances in recent years in the skin lightening area. **Chromobright®** (Dimethylmethoxy Chromanyl Palmitate) has shown to be a more effective tyrosinase inhibitor than both MAP and Arbutin, rivaling the performance of hydroquinone. **SymWhite®** (Phenylethyl Resorcinol) from pine, is considered one of the more effective natural skin lighteners in Asian countries, often used to effectively brighten intimate areas.

MITF (Microphthalmia-Associated Transcription Factor)

Research published in the last 10 years shows that MITF appears to be at the heart of a regulatory network of transcription factors and signaling pathways that control the survival, proliferation, and differentiation of melanoblasts and melanocytes. Not only is melanocyte development affected by this protein, but also pigmentation via its transcriptional regulatory effect on tyrosinase. MITF was shown to be a critical transcription factor for a key protein in melanosome transport. Therefore, MITF plays a central role in melanin synthesis, as well as melanosome biogenesis, transport, and transfer to the keratinocyte.

β-White™ (Oligopeptide-68) is a highly effective ingredient that works on the MITF pathway. This technology is unique and a boon to an industry working steadily to find a separate mechanism from the traditional lighteners.

Hormonal stimulators

There are number of hormonal stimulators of melanogenesis, known as *paracrine stimulators*. Many of them are controlled by a large hormone called *proopiomelanocortin* (POMC). Its derivatives include *α-MSH* (alpha-melanin stimulating hormone), *β-MSH*, and *ACTH*, all of which play key roles in the formation of melanin. POMC expression in keratinocytes is induced by UV. The effect of these hormones on melanogenesis has been shown with systemic administration of α-MSH, improving pigmentation predominantly in sun-exposed areas, primarily the face. The POMC peptide exerts its effect through binding what are called G-proteins to the melanocortin receptor 1 (MC1R). This intracellular second messenger is known to help regulate melanogenesis. Stimulation of specific G-protein-coupled receptors leads to the activation of *adenylyl cyclase* (AC). AC produces cAMP, which consequently stimulates the melanogenic pathway. In turn, MITF efficiently activates the melanogenetic enzyme genes such as tyrosinase and others.

Sepiwhite® (Undecylenoyl Phenylalanine) is a compound that includes amino acids and lipid residue. It has an affinity for the MC1R receptor and has been shown to inhibit melanotropin, a melanin stimulator involved in this pathway, creating a profound lightening effect beyond traditional lighteners.

Binding of a-MSH to the MC1-Receptor on melanocytes is one of the first steps in melanogenesis and pigment formation. By binding the MC1-R, we can slow the intracellular melanogenesis pathway and decrease the synthesis or the over-expression of melanin produced by melanocytes.

Melanostatine®5 (Nonapeptide-1) is a biomimetic peptide antagonist with a high affinity for MC1-R, specific to the a-MSH.

As an antagonist, Melanostatine®5 competes against the natural ligands (a-MSH) on its specific receptor (MC1-R) by preventing any further activation of the tyrosinase, thus blocking melanin synthesis.

Even though the POMC peptides have an important effect on human skin color, there are other paracrine factors that are of great importance for skin pigmentation such as endothelin-1, stem cell factor, prostaglandins, and catecholamines, to mention a few.

Melanosome transfer inhibitors

Niacinamide (vitamin B3, nicotinamide, 3-pyridinecarboxamide) is a biologically active form of niacin found in many root vegetables and yeast. Niacinamide has many cosmetic applications and roles within the skin, including increased intercellular lipid synthesis. Topical niacinamide is shown to have several benefits on aging skin, including, but not limited to, improved barrier function, improved appearance of photoaged facial skin (texture, hyperpigmentation, redness, fine lines, and wrinkles), and reduced sebum production. Additionally, niacinamide is believed to influence cutaneous pigmentation by down-regulating transfer of melanosomes from the melanocytes to the keratinocytes, although the actual process is not fully understood. Studies suggest that niacinamide has no effect on tyrosinase activity, melanin synthesis, or melanocyte number in a monolayer culture system.

In our culture, hyperpigmentation irregularities continue to be a major source of client concern. The time has never been better for skincare professionals to bring the best possible solutions to men and women at all stages of life. By staying informed and gaining experience with evolving techniques, esthetic practitioners serve as the key to a health and wellness team in providing individuals with the best corrective and preventive care. Researchers are learning and sharing more about how and why we age with the formulators seeking ever-more effective and safe products.

That, after all, is the objective of the esthetics community.

For more information on product-neutral educational classes, see the schedule at www.circadia.com

Hearing, V.J. Unraveling the melanocyte. *Am. J. Hum. Genet.* **52**(1), 1–7 (1993).

Hu, Z.M., Zhou, Q., Lei, T.C., Ding, S.F. and Xu, S.Z. Effects of hydroquinone and its glucoside derivatives on melanogenesis and antioxidation: Biosafety as skin whitening agents. J. *Dermatol.* Sci. **55**(3), 179–184 (2009)

Marles, L.K., Peters, E.M., Tobin, D.J., Hibberts, N.A. and Schallreuter, K.U. Tyrosine hydroxylase isoenzyme I is present in human melanosomes: a possible novel function in pigmentation. *Exp. Dermatol.* **12**(1), 61–70 (2003).

Boissy, R.E., Visscher, M. and DeLong, M.A. DeoxyArbutin: a novel reversible tyrosinase inhibitor with effective *in vivo* skin lightening potency. *Exp. Dermatol.* **14**(8), 601–608 (2005).

Mechanisms Regulating Skin Pigmentation: The Rise and Fall of Complexion Coloration Jody P. Ebanks, R. Randall Wickett and Raymond E. Boissy

The melanogenesis and mechanisms of skin-lightening agents – existing and new approaches

J. M. Gillbro M. J. Olsson25 January 2011

About Michael Q. Pugliese

Michael Q. Pugliese, LE (Pennsylvania) is the CEO of Circadia by Dr. Pugliese, Inc. In 2006, Michael took over the signature professional skin treatment line founded by his grandfather, Peter T. Pugliese, MD, beloved educator and author of Advanced Professional Skin Care, Medical Edition. For twelve years, Michael has continued the family tradition of educating esthetic practitioners with product-neutral lectures, covering topics of functional ingredients, cosmetic chemistry, skin physiology and disorders, and the biology of circadian rhythms. Michael's dedication and leadership have positioned Circadia as a superior education-driven American skin care company with international recognition, opening distribution in Europe, Asia, Australia, Scandinavia, Russia, and Latin America. Understanding and utilizing physiologically compatible products, Circadia by Dr. Pugliese gives estheticians tools to design effective skincare protocols for every client's concern.

Michael, member of the Society of Cosmetic Chemists, continues to investigate cutting-edge raw materials, and new product development for face and body care.

Contact info: Circadia by Dr. Pugliese, Inc Corporate Office (717) 933-2065

michael@circadia.com

Chapter 10

Make Me Be-U-tiful!!

Authored by Tina Abnoosi

The beauty industry has grown in recent years to include treatments well beyond the original tasks by cosmetic surgeons, beauticians, and aestheticians. Today, makeup artists, lash extenders, wax gurus, tattoo artists, and many others have joined this growing industry to support the evolving and growing demands of clients. Client demands are unified across the globe as everyone yearns to look younger, refreshed, and more beautiful. Understanding the depth of this desire and extent of client commitment can help us reconsider our protocols. We also need to evaluate positive interactions of modalities and procedures that may help us support and grow our business while meeting the expectations of clients.

Knowledge of appropriate skincare products and available modalities that can treat different skin conditions is essential for any provider. A modality that is very close to my heart is Microcurrent; it has consistently resulted in the reversal of the aging process by boosting the body's own healing system.

What is Microcurrent?

Microcurrent is a well-known treatment modality that has found its way back to our market. Many aestheticians and cosmetologists are rediscovering the non-invasive healing properties and numerous benefits of this modality. Microcurrent is a form of electrical massage that stimulates the skin and facial muscles without pain or adverse side effects. It is a subsensory application, so the client does not experience twitching or undesirable sensations. This modality leads to the re-education of muscles and the rebuilding of skin integrity, resulting in the disappearance of fine lines, softening of deep wrinkles, decrease in inflammation, and skin rejuvenation. Microcurrent helps cells release toxins, therefore, it's a great modality for acne treatment. It increases blood flow and establishes a healthier environment within the body to reach its homeostasis. This results in a fresh, youthful appearance. With new advancements in Microcurrent technology, its application can be easy to learn and apply, yielding results in a fraction of the time. This modality is making it possible to offer holistic treatments and meet client expectations with a noninvasive, results-oriented method.

A few noticeable outcomes of Microcurrent include:

- Reduction of dark circles and other skin discoloration.

- Decrease in puffiness and bags under eyes.

- Improvements in the appearance of fine lines, wrinkles, and sagging skin.

- Firm, lifted, and toned skin.

- Brightened skin.

- Increase of elastin and collagen with prolonged use, reducing deep lines.

Microcurrent is not for everyone!

Some contraindications that one should be aware of include:

- DO NOT use on clients who are pregnant.

- DO NOT use if client has medical electrical implants.

- DO NOT use on clients with seizure disorders.

- DO NOT use on clients with present skin cancer.

You may want to read volume one of this book for a better understanding of how Microcurrent can help in an aesthetic setting. Let's elaborate on how this modality can help other aspects of the beauty industry to make its use more prevalent among beauty professionals.

Electrified Makeovers

We use makeup to hide imperfections, contour, and highlight

facial features. Makeup is also beneficial because it allows us to express creativity, feel good about our appearance, and lift our moods. Makeup pros know that the best applications and most appealing looks start with healthy skin. Even the best homecare products and primers may fail if makeup pros do not have a truly healthy and radiant canvas to initiate work on.

Makeup artists and makeover professionals can tap into the benefits of microcurrent and allow it to deliver better results. Adding Microcurrent can accentuate facial features to significantly improve the client's look with lasting results. If you want to improve your makeup game, consider this often-underutilized-but-ever-so-versatile tool that can turn back time in the treatment room and provide quick fixes prior to application of makeup.

Microcurrent can help erase fine lines, relax over-worked muscles, and reduce puffiness and inflammation. Therefore, it can be utilized as a clearing, smoothing, lifting, defining, and contouring applicator to enhance key facial features. Microcurrent transforms and amplifies natural beauty, offering a clean canvas for the dramatic effects of follow-up makeup. The results last for a few days, giving you the confidence to look beautiful even without makeup!

Tattoo artists can benefit from the application of microcurrent because it can help reduce inflammation, support the healing of the treatment area, and seal the region of needling. This type of application therefore reduces the risk of infection.

Upper lip and eyebrow waxing are among the treatments that require special timing due to the redness. The use of Microcurrent before treatment can yield in tighter skin which reduces the risk of skin lifting. After treatment, it can help with healing and reducing redness.

The application of microcurrent has become easier as technology has advanced, making it possible and affordable to simply add a two to five-minute mini-application to a treatment. There are three simple moves that can be followed to lengthen stressed muscles, strengthen loose skin and muscles, and define important outlines of facial areas. A quick illustration of each move is shown below. Following these simple moves will result in lifting the eyelid, removing inflammation, reducing puffiness under the eye, contouring the face, or augmenting lips. These important steps share the same principle.

In applications like bridal makeovers, a minimum of two treatments within the final week can help reduce the sign of stress and provide relief as the wedding day draws near. Acne and blemishes can subside as microcurrent helps the body remove toxins and expedite the healing process.

In the more general fight against aging, many options are available before one must reach out for an invasive treatment. Let's give Microcurrent a try. Microcurrent is a silent partner that can easily help rejuvenate depleted energy without causing trauma to the body. It has no downtime and is completely sun-safe.

This modality can help in the treatment room depending on how well it is understood. The key to success is to believe in the services you offer. Taking time to evaluate Microcurrent effects on yourself and/or a few loyal clients will help you gain trust and confidence. After seeing results and the delivery you envisioned, you will realize the ease of this modality's implementation.

Microcurrent has become the most sought-after treatment by both practitioners and clients. As more people learn about the benefits of Microcurrent, the demand for the treatment will increase. The age management capability of Microcurrent can't go without notice. The re-education and maintenance of such treatment can guarantee returning clients. You may consider adopting TAMA's exclusive treatments "5 Minute Eye Lift," "Hangover Be-Gone," "Lip Augmentation in 3," and "Kissable Lips" as standalone services, add-ons, or as part of makeover treatment. The more natural and holistic remedies you offer, the healthier your clients will become. It is for certain that they will remember not only how beautiful you made them look, but how great you made them feel, ensuring their return and subsequent referrals.

Be-U-tiful!

Tina Abnoosi

President/CEO of TAMA Research Corp.

About Tina Abnoosi

Tina Abnoosi is CEO and President of TAMA Research. She holds an Electrical Engineering degree and aesthetic license with over 27 years of experience in design and manufacturing of electromagnetic components and 15 years of electro therapy (Microcurrent treatment).

She believes in USA manufacturing capabilities and supports the local businesses. Her commitment is to her customers to provide state of the art quality equipment, training and support.

Please contact Tina at (602) 354-8185 or send her an email at tina@tamaresearch.com.

Chapter 11

Mechanical Exfoliation

Authored by Mary Nielsen

Microdermabrasion is considered an essential service in an aesthetician's treatment repertoire. Minimally invasive, microdermabrasion works well as a stand-alone treatment and when integrated into a more extensive treatment plan for a client. Increasingly, clients are starting to request infused microdermabrasion treatments, typically named after specific brands such as Silk Peel, Hydrafacial, and Dermasweep.

The aspects of dry microdermabrasion are discussed here as well as an overview of infused microdermabrasion treatments.

Dry microdermabrasion can involve two different approaches. One device streams tiny aluminum oxide or other abrasive crystals across the skin. An attached vacuum simultaneously sucks the crystals back into a holding tank in the device, along with dead skin cells of the stratum corneum that have been 'sandblasted' from the surface. A second approach uses a wand that is moved across the skin. The wand tip has interchangeable grit sizes to affect the aggressiveness of the exfoliation.

Client Consultation: The consultation is intended to interview the client and find out his/her skin care goals. Removing layers of the stratum corneum can enhance the results of other treatments as well as the results of topical skin care products. The treatment has 'no down-time' and is often touted as a lunch time procedure.

Indications and Contraindications: Indications for mechanical exfoliation are varied and an assessment of the client's skin condition must be done to ascertain the client is an appropriate candidate for treatment. An improvement in fine lines and texture, an improvement in hyperpigmentation, and a reduction in breakouts are all realistic expectations after a mechanical exfoliation session.

Poor cell turnover, anti-aging concerns, acne, and superficial scarring are also reasons for a mechanical exfoliation treatment. An infused microdermabrasion will inject serums into the skin while exfoliating. Various serums can be infused based on the skin analysis. Often hydrating serums containing hyaluronic acid are used in anti-aging treatments. Salicylic acid serums are used for acne treatments. A variety of brightening agents are used to treat hyperpigmentation.

Consumer demand is high for mechanical exfoliation but it is imperative that a skin evaluation and assessment be performed to determine if there are any contraindications. Reasons to forego a treatment include active rosacea, fragile capillaries, open lesions, herpes or cold sores, warts, dermatitis or skin infection, and recent use of Vitamin A products.

Treatment: The client should sign an informed consent to treatment form. Expectations should be reviewed and the client should have the opportunity to ask questions. Photos should be taken pre-treatment. With gloves on, you should thoroughly cleanse the skin. If you are using a device with granules instead of a diamond-tip wand, the client should remove his/her contact lenses and wear protective goggles to avoid the risk of scratching the cornea from stray granules.

Section the face into smaller treatment areas. Adjust the vacuum and the flow of solution with an infused system by putting your thumb over the open tip to determine the flow of serum. Treating small sections of the face and moving systematically to cover the entire face is best. If skin laxity is present, use your non-dominant hand to hold the skin taut, which will provide a better treatment with less negative side effects such as striations on the face from skin lifting. Perform three passes on the same area. Perform each pass in a different direction on the skin; in vertical, horizontal, and diagonal directions before moving to the next area on the face. Thinner skin may need fewer passes and thicker skin may require more.

Treatments typically take 20 to 30 minutes.

Apply a hydrating serum or moisturizer and a mineral-based SPF.

When performing a microdermabrasion on a non-facial part of the body, it's important to understand that the face heals faster and more predictably than the body. The chest and neck require more healing time and should be done with lower vacuum and lighter grit.

Side Effects and Complications: The client should feel some scratching during the treatment. During infused microdermabrasion, the solution may feel cool to the skin. Mild erythema post treatment is common. The client's skin may feel sensitive but should not feel pain. Skin lifting from the vacuum could cause 'hickies' or petechiae. Superficial abrasions from faulty diamond tips with small particles that protrude are rare. Activation of the herpes virus and cold sores should be avoided by having the client pre-medicate with an antiviral.

Post Treatment: The client must keep his/her skin protected with SPF. The client can resume a skin care regimen with active ingredients (Vitamin A, glycolics) around Day 4 to Day 7. Clients will be sensitive to the sun and should avoid sun exposure.

Documentation: Documentation should include the client's skin condition pre-treatment, the grit determination, the type of infusion solution used, and application of skin care after the treatment. The client's response to the treatment, post-care instructions, the aesthetician's signature, and date should also be charted.

Safety and Sanitation: The filter in the diamond tip microdermabrasion machine should be disposed of in a sanitary manner. The device should be wiped down with the state- approved appropriate disinfectant solution. If using a crystal machine, the contents in the holding container should be disposed of in a biohazard container. For an infused device, a disinfecting solution should be used to thoroughly cleanse the tubing. Sediment and debris from dead skin cells and solution can plug tubing if not purged immediately after a treatment.

About Mary Nielsen

A technician, educator, mentor and business owner, Mary Nielsen has been at the forefront of the developments in medical esthetics since its infancy in the early 1990s. A nurse by training and experience, Mary was drawn into advanced medical esthetics with the advent of laser technologies and their use while working for a plastic surgeon. She went on to found her own successful skin and laser clinic. She is currently Vice Chair and Industry Expert on the Oregon Board of Certified Advanced Estheticians. She is the author of the advanced aesthetic textbook, A Compendium for Advanced Aesthetics, a Guide for the Master Esthetician, four books on medical spa policies and procedures, and safety policy and procedures as well as several articles on specific treatments in Skin Inc and Day Spa magazine. She is a contributor to Milady Standard Esthetics: Fundamentals, Edition 12 and writes regularly for Milady Pro.

She is the Executive Director of Spectrum Advanced Aesthetics, founder of Cascade Aesthetic Alliance, Educational Catalyst for Skintelligent Resources, and owner of Indie Aesthetics.

Contact Mary Today!

Email: mary@spectrumlasertraining.com

Chapter 12

What's Been Missing in our Treatment Rooms: Acoustic Resonance

Authored by Mary Schook

As I board my flight to Tokyo, I ponder my curse of insatiable thirst for discovering and formulating magical beauty solutions to help enhance the world. It's an addiction I will never be able to cure.

AESTHETIC TRENDS THAT LED ME TO ACOUSTIC RESONANCE

LASH EXTENSIONS

Everyone asks me "how did you get here." I won't bore you with the detours and stops along the journey through aesthetics, but there were some important highlights. It all began when lashes chose me. As a makeup artist, I was already creating lashes for fashion editorials, ad campaigns, and the NY, Milan, and Paris runways. It was necessary to introduce exciting, alternative materials to remain fashion forward.

Lash extensions became my first major beacon heard around the globe, thanks to the captivating article by Vogue's contributing editor Marina Rust, the polishing touches by Beauty Editor Sarah Brown, and the blessings of Editor in Chief Anna Wintour. A license for extensions didn't even exist back then, and the only resources were DVD's in Korean (if you could find a player) until Lavish Lashes created the first training program. The article came in perfect time, resulting in 100+ customers ringing my phone each day for nearly a month. But the real catalyst/instigator for which I will forever be grateful is the legendary fashion hair stylist Orlando Pita. We can all thank him for nudging me front and center of the beauty world. He intuitively knew that women (and some men) needed lashes and we've never looked back in the U.S., even over fifteen years later!

STEM CELLS AND GROWTH FACTORS

At the turn of the century, stem cell growth factors were a brief craze in cosmetic and aesthetic services. A medical lab in South Korea originated and released the most brilliant stem cell media product. The growth factors remained freeze-dried in an airless chamber contained inside a second serum ampoule. It wasn't until the customer activated the serum with a pump, thereby mixing the delivery system with the media, that the "cells" (growth factors) activated. As long as the customer used the refrigerated ampoule within the week, it was guaranteed viable. It was a $2,000 system, but the results were remarkable and it was a major catalyst behind the future Korean Beauty Wave.

Stem cell growth factors never quite gained traction because the labs were inconsistent with the media and their outcome can be quite unpredictable (at a great expense to both the practitioner and the consumer). A majority of the stem cell growth factor companies are now a memory. Sadly, most of what remains is only marketing, whether the source is Porcine (pig), Bovine (cow), Ovine (sheep), Plant, Embryonic, Adipose, or any other Human-derived cell. If the "stem cells" or "growth factors" were in fact viable, they would still lose their optimum usage during formulation, transportation, or administration.

KOREAN BEAUTY WAVE

The South Korean Stem Cell Media product's results caught the attention of contributing beauty editor Courtney Dunlop. With great enthusiasm, Courtney whispered into Marie Claire Beauty Editor Ying Chu's ear about a land far across the ocean called South Korea. It was no longer a third-world country and the South Korean government was funding businesses to disrupt the entire beauty industry, using cute packaging and functional cosmetics (that [once] lived up to their claims at over a fourth of the price of their competitors). We no longer had to buy a $200 or $450 cream hoping to see results. Aside from the $2,000 stem cell kit, $20 was enough to buy clinically-proven transformation for your skin. Consumers wanted to see some kind of benefit from relinquishing their hard-earned cash for more hope in a jar. Sephora, Ulta, Target, Urban Outfitters, and other retailers are taking advantage of this while they still can (despite China's economic hit to South Korea, curtailing the country's innovation and production).

ENTER SOUND THERAPY

I feel the most important introduction of my career has been patented sound technology from Asia. Sound Technology goes by many names, but in the treatment room, we call this Acoustic Resonance. AR is low-level sound that creates a very specific, controlled vibration that resides in a spectrum below Ultrasound (medical) and above Infrasound (invisible sound). The vibration is audible to the human ear. If you've ever pressed up against a speaker playing music, you've felt a vibration emitting from the sound coming through the speakers. This is the sensation I'm referring to when discussing AR.

This entry is not about educating you on the "science" of Acoustic Resonance. AR/Vibroacoustic "Technology" sounds like pseudoscience (especially when it pertains to tuning forks and singing bowls). While those modalities may have been around for thousands of years, AR is rather new and has yet to be proven in serious medical journals.

WE ARE VIBRATION

On a cellular level, human beings also vibrate. The effects of sound can be physiological, psychological, and neurological depending on the sound and its delivery. These kinds of vibrations can only be seen through a special microscope. MIT researchers state "a red blood cell has electrical, chemical, and biological activity taking place inside it, which causes nanoscale vibrations at its surface." "To establish the connection between the cells' vibration and their health, the researchers used Feld's technique to create three-dimensional images" of this vibration. (1)

Even noted scientists and inventors like Albert Einstein and Nikola Tesla said over a century ago that we are vibration. Tesla stated, "If you want to find the secrets of the universe, think in terms of energy, frequency, and vibration."(2) Tesla was so far advanced in his thinking. In aesthetics, we have never truly broached vibration.

WHAT HARMS OUR VIBRATION

As we go through life, vibrations change or are disrupted by negative vibrations such as EMF waves, low energy foods, toxic products, stress, and a toxic environment. Low vibration can result in fatigue, negativity, physical illness, or inflammation. In skincare, it can lead to aging, inflammation, dry skin, lack of elasticity, and more.

VIBRATION IS NOT NEW

As I mentioned earlier, Sound Therapy is not new. It has been used for thousands of years by various cultures for healing and restoring harmony in the body and cells depending on the sound's delivery. Those sounds may elevate or transport us, but try balancing a singing bowl on your knee or forehead.

As aestheticians, we know that delivery is crucial. You can have the best ingredients in a jar, but unless you have the right ingredients with correct delivery, you're only wasting good money on ingredients flooding already dead skin. The same concept of delivery applies to sound.

I've had the chance to research and experience a LOT of the latest Vibroacoustic technology. I've tried beds, audio programs, chairs, mats, tables, devices that look like Russian military stim machines, and much more. During my experiences, I either could not reach a relaxed state or the modalities would cause undesired outcomes. It's difficult to create and match the perfect sound sequence or harmony for the body, especially because our brainwaves are all unique.

AR IN MEDICAL

The medical side of AR is still being studied for stem cell growth, joint pain, neurological conditions, and various illnesses. Vibroacoustic Therapy "pioneer" Olav Skille, alternative doctors, and researchers are still trying to connect specific sounds to specific issues to benefit the body. The proof of sound therapy efficacy has a LONG way to go.

"AMP"LIFYING AESTHETICS

Applying AR to aesthetics and massage helps us achieve results faster within the scope of our practices. When we choose to administer sound to customers during lymphatic drainage or massages, we are "amp"lifying their results.

Like in the medical world, aestheticians are in the beginnings of collecting data on Acoustic services. The device introduced during Shelley Hancock's Show and Tell, which is used by aestheticians and massage therapists, is not a medical device. It is a technology inspired by other pioneers in the sound field, resulting in the sculpting of the face, skin tightening, and deep relaxation of the body. When combining AR with other modalities such as microcurrent, one can render youthful, long-lasting, and cumulative results, leaving the client in a very relaxed state.

BEWARE OF VIBRATION

I want to emphasize that there are a lot of devices that claim to be AR. Vibration can be created by a motor, not by sound, making it enormously different from AR. Vibration can be destructive and cause problems on the surface of the skin. AR can either be gentle surface vibration or deep therapeutic massage. It's the same as comparing a heating pad that only heats the surface of the skin, to a long-wave infrared pad that can penetrate up to eight inches into the body. One pad can burn you at the skin's surface while the other can enhance your skin.

THANK YOU

I hope I've enlightened you about a new modality that will soon become essential to every treatment room across the globe. Sound has always been here and is not going anywhere......and we're so addicted!

1. Vibrating Cells Disclose Their Ailments. Michael Fitzgerald. 09/09/08

https://www.technologyreview.com/s/410793/vibrating-cells-disclose-their-ailments/

2. Wikipedia- Nikola Tesla

About Mary Schook

Mary Schook® has been at the forefront of the intersection of beauty and well-being for more than 20 years as a New York-based licensed aesthetician, cosmetic formulator, and owner of Beauty By Mary Schook, LLC and its various enterprises.

Mary is a rich source of beauty expertise and cutting-edge breakthroughs for editors and their readers, which is why she is consistently featured on the pages of American Vogue, Allure, the New York Times, Marie Claire, New York Magazine, People, Cosmopolitan, Refinery 29, and countless other periodicals while making appearances on NBC, Bravo, Rachael Ray, and various media platforms.

Mary Schook is also constantly introducing new products and innovations to buyers and professionals across the globe to help them differentiate their customer offerings- a major factor in the popularization of Korean beauty products pioneered by Schook.

"Beauty's Mad Scientist"- Vogue

"Christopher Columbus to Korea's New World"- Marie Claire

Chapter 13

The New Brow

Authored by Jaclyn Peresetsky

Eyebrow shape is unarguably one of the most important facial features and has become the superstar feature. Squared, rounded, thick, thin, long, or arched, brow shapes and sizes are endless. Brow products are flying off the shelves as everyone seems to be filling or darkening their brows to improve or enhance their shape. Images on Instagram, Facebook, and Pinterest make perfect brows seem effortless, giving all users brow envy! By now, everyone is acutely aware that brows are what truly frame the face. It's no surprise that brow treatments and services are on the rise, and clients are seeking a way to have the perfect brow.

Trends may come and go, but inevitably, the fuller, thicker brow is in demand. Those who have over-tweezing regrets or a naturally thinning brow are starting to consider a longer lasting option over drawing their brows on every day. Permanent makeup may have been a bit too daunting for most, so interestingly, a new brow service has emerged. Microblading eyebrows first rose to prominence about 25 years ago throughout Asia. Its history is not well-documented in the U.S., and it doesn't help that it's gone by so many different names: microstroking, feather tattooing, eyebrow tattooing, "the Japanese Method," feathering, hairstroking, etc. In Asia, the technique matured as artists experimented with different brow patterns, tools, and application techniques. A lot of modern techniques are now taken for granted and commonplace. Originally, many artists would cross hairstrokes in an "x" pattern, since real hairs do cross. However, this would injure the skin and look less natural. These days, most artists are taught never to cross hairstrokes.

Today, more advanced techniques such as "3D Eyebrows" are popular throughout the United States. Newer techniques are still being innovated in Asia, such as the "6D Eyebrow" by artists like David Zhang. In the last few years, microblading has had a surge of popularity throughout Europe, where schools and artists have established themselves as the frontier of microblading for the West. This less permanent option seems to be more appealing to some. Microblading is a good option for those who want to fully reconstruct, define, fill in gaps, or redefine over-tweezed brows with less commitment. Many clients have a naturally straighter brow, but an arch makes them look younger later in life. Those who are interested in microblading like the crisper, more natural hair stroke of a brow rather than some traditional permanent brow options. Although, both microblading and permanent makeup have hair stroke techniques available. Ultimately, those who love microblading do not want to commit to a specific brow shape because of changes in personal appearance or trends. As a permanent makeup artist, I have seen opportunities for merging permanent makeup techniques and microblading techniques.

The Microblading Procedure

In general, a topical numbing cream is applied prior to any permanent makeup or microblading procedure to minimize client's discomfort. Everyone has a different pain and anxiety tolerance, so it is important to get a feel for your clients at the time of consultation, especially if you have never done a service on them before. Always have them fill out new paperwork designed specifically for microblading beforehand. During a consult, you can also pre-discuss design, shape, and color, as well as patch test and take before pictures.

What is Microblading?

Microblading is when you use a hand-held tool comprised of 6-14 micro-needles in the shape of a blade (hence the name microblade) to make micro-slices in the skin. The technique is to drag the needle with a tiny amount of pigment, mimicking a hair stroke. Then, follow by re-dipping the needle tip and adding pigment carefully into the slice with the microblade. This technique allows the skin to heal with a fine and crisp hair stroke, much like real hair. The slice must carefully reach the upper dermis, which is very challenging because you need to sense what layer you are in. Throughout the procedure, the pigment is continuously rubbed on top to help push pigment into the skin to reach the right layer. The technician will create a strategic hair pattern to emulate a natural brow. There is a lot of thought and pre-planning that goes into studying the natural brow hair pattern. This pattern is where the difficulty in the procedure comes into play. Microblading is extremely technical and detailed because each hair stroke must be purposeful. Proper lighting, such as a head lamp, is crucial, along with having plenty of time, approximately 2 hours, for the initial procedure. Microblading typically lasts 12-18 months and refreshers are recommended as the pigment fades.

Permanent makeup techniques differ because they use a rotary device such as a pen machine to implant pigment into the upper layer of the dermis. The device's motion is similar to a vibrating sewing needle motion. The machine's strength allows the pigment to be deposited strategically at a particular depth through a particular technique. There are different needle tips that can be attached to the machine's hand piece that allow for different shapes and techniques; this can include powder brow, shading, hairstrokes, or a fusion. One of the major differences from microblading is that the machine's vibration in permanent makeup may cause the hairstroke to "blur" or soften. However, there are new needle tips known as micros that emulate the microblade stroke, but with more permanency. Permanent makeup lasts 3-5 years and refreshers are recommended as the pigment fades.

Who is a microblading candidate?

Determining candidates for microblading can be a bit more challenging as it truly depends on the integrity and quality of the skin. Most often, you see pictures online of "before and after" results that are not necessarily true. Technicians post right after the procedure to claim perfect work when the image is not the actual healed result. In fact, like most permanent makeup procedures, microblading needs 2-3 applications of color to ensure enough color holds. A good way to tell if the picture was taken immediately after a procedure is if the newly done brows have a yellow halo effect. This results from the epinephrine in the anesthetic that constricts capillaries and lessens bleeding during the procedure. Another important factor is that microblading "after" pictures are of those with perfectly smooth skin. This is because those who have skin that is too thin or heavily textured are not great candidates for microblading. In fact, the micropigmentation industry has done a great job in categorizing skin into food types, so there is a universal understanding of the skin types that are good candidates and the skin types that are not. For example, microblading slices the skin by dragging a blade and implanting pigment. The pigment is deposited in the upper dermis and is visible through the skin. Whatever textures or irregularities of the dermis and epidermis will affect how the pigment looks (i.e. crooked hair strokes or blotchy and uneven color). Case in point, skin types that are thin, oily, heavily lined, wrinkled, and have large pores are not suitable for microblading. A permanent makeup option would be better for these skin types because the machine offers multiple techniques that allow an even distribution of pigment with softer shading effects.

A good technician should have a lot of experience with pigment color and an understanding of how it heals in the skin. Often, this is the most difficult thing to master in microblading or permanent makeup. The same pigments that are used for permanent makeup are used for microblading. There are many factors to consider in color choice: skin color and undertone, skin integrity, skin health, internal chemistry of the body, and pigment color and undertone. I have an advanced art education as well as a specialty degree in color, and it took me years to understand the complexity of implanting color into the skin. As a makeup artist, I struggled with understanding the relation of color implanted INTO skin and color topically applied ONTO skin. I utilized my knowledge of color chemistry, color theory, and color relationships when I had difficulty grasping the concept. You can select five people and use the same color on all five but get different results. Some clients will hold on to pigment easily while others won't. In addition, you may need to change up your pigment choice or technique after observing initial healing. Some will heal too cool (grey, blue or purple undertone), too light, or too dark. A touchup is when you tweak the color or application technique based on the healed result. It takes time and experience to learn how color works in the skin as well as what technique suits each specific skin type.

Expectations after Microblading

Every technician's post-care recommendations will vary, but for the most part, the goal is to keep the procedure area clean and dry. To protect the area from harmful bacteria or environmental aggressors, the client is typically sent out the door with grapeseed oil or ointment applied to the brows and post-care instructions. Immediately after procedure, the treated area needs to be protected from harmful bacteria and environmental aggressors. Over the next few days, the brows will slightly crust and flake as the skin layers heal underneath. If clients pull or pick at the crust, they can lift the pigment. You must be a cheerleader and encourage your clients to resist the temptation. Clients should not work out, sweat, or take hot steamy showers a few days following the procedure. They should also avoid planning big events until after their touchups are complete. The touchups can be done between 4-6 weeks after the initial procedure. Over time, the pigment naturally exfoliates, lightens, and fades. Sun exposure or tanning beds and active skincare products such as hydroquinone and retinols will fade pigment much faster. Also, an inexperienced technician may not have applied the pigment deep enough into the skin, which usually results in much faster fading.

The Future of Microblading

Because microblading is a newer procedure, we will continue to learn more about how the brows should be maintained after long periods of fading or after multiple touchups and/or refreshers since delicate hair strokes can be easily skewed. Also, we will learn more about new techniques for implanting colors as newer tools and pigments are continuously created. Recently, technicians have started to add shading with the microblade hand tool or rotary machine to soften hair strokes and add more dimension. This technique seems to work well for clients who hardly have brows at all; those who have an obvious stop in brow hair or more mature brows that need softness and lifting. This is truly my favorite technique because powder shading fills brows with makeup, which adds beautiful depth and alleviates any hollow sections while maintaining naturally sweeping hair strokes. I also think this technique will be easier to maintain over time.

Whether you are considering learning microblading or you have already begun, know that like esthetics, it is an ongoing journey and learning process. As time goes on, you will get better and better. Be patient with yourself. Make sure to check with the American Academy of Micropigmentation to ensure the trainer or facility you choose is reputable because you will need ongoing training and mentorship. It is best to learn from those who are true pros in the industry so they can help you get through challenging procedures and complex color decisions. With every newer technique like microblading, sharing experiences will always allow us to rise to new challenges and improve each procedure along the bright new path.

About Jaclyn Peresetsky

Jaclyn Peresetsky is not only the owner of Skin Perfect Spas in Ohio and Florida, but she is also a noted color expert, makeup artist, master esthetician, permanent makeup instructor, author, and speaker. Her multiple books, cosmetic and skin care lines, and training courses allow other beauty pros to learn and add more services that combine art and science to become leading beauty experts. Her passion for education led her to create a school for Advanced Esthetics and Color, opening in January of 2019 in Columbus, OH.

Contact Info:

Jaclyn Peresetsky

Owner of Skin Perfect Spas & Colore Me Perfect Cosmetics

www.skinperfectclinic.com

www.coloremeperfect.com

Office: 239-262-5110

jaclyn@skinperfectclinic.com

Chapter 14

Ultrasonic Skin Spatula, AKA Skin Scrubber

Authored by Beatrice Van

Let's talk about one of my favorite devices. An oldie, but a newbie…The Ultrasonic Skin Spatula also known as the Skin Scrubber! This device emits high frequency sonic waves, which provide facial treatments that cleanse, exfoliate, repair, and stimulate the skin. This device is based on high frequency mechanical oscillations produced by the metal spatula-like tool. The scrubber vibrates up to 30,000 Hz. The oscillation is created through a water medium which makes it an effective device for removing dead skin cells and other impurities from the skin.

The Ultrasonic Skin Scrubber has been proven to offer several benefits including, but not limited to:

- Reducing clogged pores and excess sebum.
- Improving skin texture.
- Scrubbing gently, but effectively, making it a suitable choice for those with sensitive skin.
- Supporting skin tightening.
- Minimizing signs of fine line and wrinkles.
- Promoting smoother and softer skin.
- Helping the penetration of skin care products.
- Improving skin circulation.

Before I share a few of my go-to skin scrubber facial protocols, here is a quick rundown on the modes. A skin spatula typically comes with two modes; Infusion Mode and Scrubber Mode.

Infusion Mode helps aid the penetration of your treatment serums and moisturizers by using the flat side of the spatula against the skin (refer to image below). You will feel the spatula gently tapping the product deep into the skin. The vibration of the scrubber will also gently massage and tone the skin while it creates a fine mist that also removes the excess water from the face during the application.

Scrubber Mode helps cleanse and exfoliate the skin. By applying the tip of the spatula at a 45-degree angle and slowly moving in a downward motion all over the treatment area, you will see the comedones and dead skin cells blast off the face. The tip of the device will also collect the comedones and dead skin cells. You should always see a consistent mist (oscillation) when using this mode for proper cleansing and exfoliation of the skin. Pro Tip: lift the skin in congested areas with your thumb and index finger "pinching" the section to put more pressure under the comedone.

A few things to consider when using the Ultrasonic Skin Scrubber:

- Be gentle, let the device do the work for you.
- Do not overuse.
- Do not use it on clients with epilepsy.
- Do not use on clients who are pregnant.

- Do not use on lesions suspicious for cancer.

- Maintain contact and do not apply pressure.

- Do not use it on cystic acne, nodular cystic acne, and small or large papules, infections, open wounds or sores.

Here are a few of my favorite go-to facial treatments with the skin spatula!!!

ANTI-AGING – BRIGHTENING FACIAL

STEP 1 – CLEANSE

Cleanse and tone the skin with appropriate cleanser and toner.

STEP 2 – EXFOLIATE

Gently exfoliate the skin with a jojoba bead scrub. Pat some water over the skin and gently remove exfoliating product with Ultrasonic Skin Spatula, tip-side down. Make sure that your spatula oscillates while it glides on top of the skin. If you do not see the mist, apply more water to the skin. Remove excess product off the tip with a clean piece of gauze, paper towel, or clean towel. Tone skin with an AHA toner.

STEP 3 – EXTRACTION

Extract any unwanted comedones from the skin. If the skin is heavily blemished, perform a second cleansing after extractions to help remove any surface bacteria. Tone the skin with appropriate toner.

STEP 4 – REVITALIZE

Apply a thin layer of a papaya enzyme mask. As you apply the mask, let your clients know that they may feel a little spicy or tingly sensation. It usually lasts about a minute or two and then subsides. If the client says the mask feels like it's "burning", remove the mask with a cool moistened towel. I would NOT apply steam or hot towel compress with this mask because it may intensify the treatment too much. Follow manufacturer's guidelines for length of time on the skin. Remove all traces of product with a cool moistened towel followed by a cool moistened gauze to your client until the itchiness or tingling sensation goes away. Tone the skin.

STEP 5 – LED LIGHT THERAPY

Using LED light therapy will stimulate fibroblasts, increasing collagen and elastin. In just minutes, you can reduce the appearance of fine lines and wrinkles, and improve skin texture, quality, and smoothness.

STEP 6A – INFUSION

Apply a quality hyaluronic acid, L-ascorbic acid to stimulate collagen, and a high peptide serum to the forehead, eye area, and lips. If you are treating hyperpigmentation, follow with a melanin inhibiting serum on targeted areas. A serum with hydroquinone will induce melanocytes-specific cytotoxicity, and Azelaic and kojic acid will help reduce the number of melanin granules and interfere with melanogenesis. During this time, you can add a light, relaxing facial or pressure point massage. Apply treatment eye cream.

STEP 6B – PENETRATION

Using the "infusion" mode on an ultrasonic skin scrubber, penetrate the amino peptide serum into the key areas of the face. The client may notice a light tingling as the product penetrates the skin.

STEP 7 – MOISTURIZE & PROTECT

Complete the treatment with a skin softening and nourishing anti-aging moisturizer, followed with a nice sun protection lotion of at least SPF 30.

CLARITY FACIAL

STEP 1 – CLEANSE

Apply appropriate cleanser to the face and make sure you foam it up with water. Set the ultrasonic skin scrubber to its "scrubber" mode. Gently remove cleanser with the ultrasonic skin spatula tip-side down. Make sure that your spatula oscillates while it glides on top of the skin. If you do not see the mist, apply more water to the skin. Remove excess product off the tip with a clean piece of gauze, paper towel, or clean towel, and then tone the skin with an AHA toner.

STEP 2 – EXTRACTION

To effectively loosen compacted sebum and help simplify the extraction process, apply a detoxifying product to impacted pores, then steam and massage the skin lightly for 3-5 minutes. Extract any unwanted comedones from the skin. If the skin is heavily blemished, perform a second cleansing after extractions to help remove any surface bacteria. Spark papules and pustules with a high frequency device. Tone the skin.

STEP 4 – REVITALIZE

Apply a thin layer of a pumpkin enzyme mask (pumpkin contains a high percentage of naturally occurring salicylic acid, which is great to treat problematic skin). As you apply the mask, let your clients know that they may feel a little spicy or tingly sensation. It usually lasts about a minute or two and then subsides. If the client says the mask feels like it's "burning", remove the mask with a cool moistened towel. I would NOT apply steam or hot towel compress with this mask because it may intensify the treatment too much. Follow manufacturer's guidelines for length of time to be left on the skin. Remove all traces of product with a cool moistened towel followed by a cool moistened gauze until your client no longer feels the itchiness or tingling sensation. Tone skin with a calming toner.

STEP 5 – CALM

Place a jade roller in a small bowl of ice. Calm the skin with an aloe-based mask. Leave on 5-7 minutes. Perform a relaxing scalp, hand, and arm, or neck and shoulder massage while the mask sits on the skin. Continue to calm the skin with cold jade rollers. Roller over skin for 3-5 minutes. Remove with a cool moistened towel or pre-moistened gauze. Tone the skin with a calming toner.

STEP 6 - LED LIGHT THERAPY

LED light therapy works safely and effectively, using no abrasive chemicals or harmful UV-rays or side effects, to destroy acne-causing bacteria — not only does it clear up existing blemishes, but it prevents future breakouts.

STEP 7A - INFUSION

Apply a niacinamide serum (vitamin B-6, which improves epidermal barrier function, reduces sebum excretion rate, and brightens), a benzoyl peroxide or salicylic acid spot treatment, and a quality hyaluronic acid to the skin. Apply treatment eye cream. Depending on the skin type, you can perform a light, relaxing facial or pressure point massage.

STEP 7B – PENETRATION

Using the "infusion" mode on an ultrasonic skin scrubber, penetrate the serums into the key areas of the face. The client may notice a light tingling as the product penetrates the skin.

STEP 8 – MOISTURIZE & PROTECT

Complete the treatment with a light weight nourishing moisturizer, followed by a nice sun protection lotion of at least SPF 30.

SOOTHING FACIAL

STEP 1 & 2 – CLEANSE & EXFOLIATE

Apply appropriate cleanser to the face and make sure you foam it up with water. Set the ultrasonic skin scrubber to its "scrubber" mode. Gently remove cleanser with ultrasonic skin spatula tip-side down. Make sure that your spatula oscillates while it glides on top of the skin. If you do not see the mist, apply more water to the skin. Remove excess product off the tip with a clean piece of gauze, paper towel, or clean towel, and then tone the skin with a soothing toner.

STEP 3 – SOOTHE

Place a jade roller in a small bowl of ice. Apply an aloe-based mask to the skin. Leave on 5-7 minutes. Apply cool pre-moistened gauze on the skin, keeping the mouth and nose exposed so the client can breathe. Perform a relaxing scalp, hand, and arm, or neck and shoulder massage while mask rests on the skin. Continue to calm the skin with cold jade rollers. Roll jade over skin for 3-5 minutes. Remove mask with pre-moistened gauze, followed by a cool moistened towel. Tone the skin with a calming toner.

STEP 4 - LED LIGHT THERAPY

This boost of cellular energy results in a cascade of metabolic events leading to an increase in micro-circulation, tissue repair, and a decrease in inflammation.

STEP 5A – INFUSION

Apply a serum containing sodium hyaluronate, which holds 1,000 times its weight in water and reduces TEWL or brisabolol (chamomile), to calm and soothe the skin while reducing visible redness or apply a serum containing retinol and niacinamide. This blend is combined with soothing and calming ingredients that reduce signs of aging, redness, and strengthen skin without irritation. Apply treatment eye cream. Depending on the skin type, perform a light, relaxing facial massage or pressure point massage.

STEP 5B – PENETRATION

Using the "infusion" mode on the ultrasonic skin scrubber, penetrate the serums into the key areas of the face. The client may notice a light tingling as the product penetrates the skin.

STEP 6 – MOISTURIZE & PROTECT

Complete the treatment with a skin soothing and nourishing moisturizer, followed by a nice sun protection lotion of at least SPF 30.

About Beatrice Van

Beatrice Van, an enthusiastic, positive self-starter, has over 16 years of progressive experience in the beauty industry. Her Clinical Master Aesthetic Students and clients call her a skin magician. In addition to her role as Clinical Master Aesthetics Educator at Spectrum Advanced Aesthetics, she's licensed in advanced aesthetics, makeup artistry, and nail technology. On her days off, she's helping brides look and feel their very best or traveling throughout North America as an Education Ambassador for CND. Being well-balanced, her roles include educator, advanced trainer, practicing spa, medi-spa, and nail specialist. Beatrice has had numerous published works from hands-on experience, including Lead Artist for both Bridal and Creative editorial makeup team. Her passion is to empower students and beauty professionals to boldly invest in their education, strengthen their skills, and elevate industry standards. For more information on her facial treatment protocols, devices, or specific products used, contact Beatrice at beatrice@spectrumlasertraining.com.

Chapter 15

Stem Cells, Growth Factors, & Cytokines in Skincare

Authored by Daniel Clary

When it comes to skin health, does the "social activity" of your skin cells ever cross your mind? In fact, were you aware that your skin even had a social life? Well-understood biology confirms that your cells have VERY active social interactions. They are constantly communicating with one another, giving off messages that instruct coordinated biological events that influence how cells function and behave. All nucleated human cells, outside of red blood cells, communicate by giving off messenger proteins called cytokines and growth factors. Each of these proteins carry a unique "instruction." Medical literature, including publications such as the Journal of Drugs in Dermatology, recognize these proteins as the molecular "keys" that unlock the full potential of your cells to stimulate and optimize skin health. As we begin to grasp the fundamentals behind aging and aging skin, we are realizing that if we don't optimize cellular communication, powerful actives in research-proven ingredients will not perform at the highest level when exposed to skin. Growth Factors and cytokines allow us to achieve this very objective. However, not all growth factors and cytokines are created equal.

Before discussing the effects of growth factors and cytokines on the skin, it is necessary to understand that it is their combined "pattern" that determines their effects (all cells secrete dozens, if not hundreds, of growth factors and cytokines.) That pattern is determined by the genetic machinery of the cells being cultured to obtain the growth factors and cytokines - most frequently stem cells from liposuction fat, stem cells from bone marrow, or fibroblasts from male infant foreskins. The role of growth factors and cytokines in healing wounds has been studied extensively; they serve multiple functions including regulating the immune system, promoting collagen synthesis, quenching inflammation, increasing inflammation, reducing scar tissue, and so on.

I want to emphasize the ability of these proteins to either INCREASE or DECREASE inflammation. This is their most important aspect when it comes to comparing the different sources of growth factors and cytokines, and ultimately, finding out what physiological effect they will have on the skin. It should come as no surprise to anyone that inflammation and aging are synonymous. Any topical product for anti-aging, in its truest sense, must be strongly anti-inflammatory.

Before I dive into the different sources of these proteins, let's briefly discuss basic "mechanism of action". As previously mentioned, these biological signals are how cells "talk" to each other. They work in sort of a "lock and key" fashion. Think of the growth factor or cytokine as the "key", and the receptor on the cell's surface as the "lock". A growth factor ("key") gets synthesized within a cell; then, the cell releases the growth factor, which travels to neighboring cells and attaches to receptors on the cells' surfaces ("lock"), activating a unique biological response. A cascade of biologic signals is sent to the heart of the cell, the nucleus, causing a change in genetic expression. The behavior of the neighboring cells changes. This process continues to complete the task at hand. This is cell-to-cell communication in its simplest explanation.

Now, let's move on to the sources of signal proteins and why they are important. The terms growth factor, cytokine, and stem cells get thrown around quite often in skin care marketing, with a ton of misinformation about what these terms actually mean. Often, the "magical" plant stem cell gets sensationalized in the skin care arena. Without spending too much time diving into this, when it comes to cell-to-cell communication within HUMAN skin, plants serve no purpose or function. It is physiologically impossible for plant stem cells to communicate with human cells; they don't speak the same language. That's not to say that they don't have some therapeutic value; research shows the potential anti-oxidant capability from certain plant species. That being said, it is vital that we expose human-derived growth factors and cytokines to the skin to achieve the physiological effect we desire.

There are hundreds of different types of growth factors and cytokines. Within the realm of human-derived growth factors, there are multiple cells we can utilize to extract powerful cellular messenger proteins. Let's first discuss the process of "extraction" to give you a better understanding. An easy way to recognize a product with human-derived protein is when the label says "_____ conditioned media", the blank space being the cell of choice. Independent of the cell used (we will discuss this next), the culturing process is as follows:

-In the lab, the cell of choice is placed into a "glorified" petri dish that contains a media solution. We like to call this a "nutrient-rich broth". This media is basically a nutritional source for the cells to feed off and grow.

-As the cells grow, they begin to replicate themselves; the number of cells exponentially increases within the culture/media.

-While growing, the cells start to give off/release their naturally produced growth factors and cytokines into the broth/media.

-Once this process is complete, the living cells are filtered out of the broth/media, and you are left with the growth factors, cytokines, enzymes, exosomes, and other material the cell released.

-The media is now "conditioned" and ready to be processed and formulated for topical application.

Barring a few additional steps that would be too technical to discuss, this is the simplified process. Depending on the cell used, each gives off a unique portfolio of proteins whose net pattern determines the physiological effect on the skin.

There are three main cell types cultured for topical application; Fibroblast cells, Adipose (Fat) Stem Cells, and Bone Marrow Stem Cells. The pattern of proteins each produces is vastly different from another.

Fibroblast Cells: Even though it is still widely used, the Fibroblast cell type is considered "first generation" growth factor skin care. Fibroblast cells are the dominant cell within connective tissue. These cells synthesize key structural protein such as collagen and elastin. When cultured (usually from neonatal tissue), they begin to release messenger bio-signals like any other cell. Fibroblasts, however, are considered "low-ranking" cells. The number of cytokines and growth factors they release into the media are minute. They are WEAK producers of bio-signals. They have some even teetering on the inflammatory side. Manufacturers will compensate for this by adding a larger dose of the media in their products. In no way does this improve efficacy; it simply makes the product stink (human protein has a distinct smell!).

Adipose (Fat) Stem Cells: Sourced from middle-aged donors and a byproduct of liposuction waste, Adipose (Fat) Stem Cells are cheap, easy to culture, and grown in abundance. The inherent problem with these cells is that they serve no role in controlled healing within the body. Fat Stem Cells have one fate in life and that is to create more fat. Fat serves auxiliary endocrine function and when these stem cells are cultured, the portfolio of proteins released into the media are strongly PRO-INFLAMMATORY.

Metabolically active hormones such as leptin, and cytokines such as TNF-a and IL-6, could disrupt healthy biochemical pathways. Remember that aging and inflammation go hand-in-hand. If the objective of a daily skin care product is anti-aging, it is strongly encouraged that you avoid using Adipose Stem Cell-derived growth factors and cytokines.

Bone Marrow Stem Cells: This cell type is the master stem cell that controls healing and regeneration throughout the entire body. In fact, it is the only MOBILE stem cell that patrols the body looking for injury. Upon discovery of that injury, it initiates a regenerative response to heal. When cultured (sourced from healthy young adult donors), bone marrow stem cells release an abundance of growth factors and cytokines that are predominantly ANTI-INFLAMMATORY and PRO-HEALING, such as TGF-b3, IGF-1, and IL-10. It is this net-pattern of protein that provides an unparalleled anti-aging response on the skin. No other cell in the body can fight inflammation quite like this cell type.

It is also important to remember that growth factors do not exist in isolation and no product should contain a single protein molecule (think of the EGF cream craze in the late nineties). You want to use a product that has a physiologically balanced composition of these proteins and has an anti-inflammatory net-pattern of bio-signals. As an aesthetic practitioner, I encourage you to dive deeper into the research of this technology and constantly ask questions about the products manufacturers are selling. Armed with this knowledge, you have the power to choose formulations that truly optimize this social network that exists within your skin and have it work with you, not against you.

Your skin is talking, are you listening?

About Daniel Clary

Daniel Clary is a passionate aesthetic industry veteran, with over 15 years as a licensed esthetician in two states. He has worked with some of the best world-class spas, skin care companies, and medical facilities, and has had his hand in product formulation, menu creation, designing protocols, and training. His entire career has been immersed in cosmetic chemistry, skin physiology, and molecular biology, learning from some of the greatest minds in the industry. He has fostered a wealth of knowledge, which has allowed him to be a keynote speaker at medical and esthetic conferences and has been published in respected journals. An elected member of the Society of Cosmetic Chemists, he strives to deliver top-notch education and is part of a team of science "truth-seekers" as VP of Education at AnteAGE. He also maintains a new beauty and science-focused blog at www.culturedbeauty.com. He currently resides in sunny Phoenix, AZ.

Chapter 16

Attracting Business

Authored by Shelley Hancock

I want to share some of the things that I feel helped me in creating my successful skincare business of 30 years. The first thing is passion. Do you love being an Esthetician? Passion for this industry is the first step to becoming successful. You can't fake it. You either have it or you don't, and those who have it will more likely be successful.

Are you having fun being an Esthetician? Are you truly having fun? If so, your business should reflect that and you should be absolutely swamped with clients. People are attracted to the energy of passion and excitement. They want to be around it. I would rather see you not know all the technical terms of this industry but have super positive energy than be extremely book savvy, touting language that the clients don't even understand with low passive energy. Clients will not be attracted to that.

When chatting with my fellow Estheticians and reading posts on the forums, I'm hearing that you are wanting very particular, exact step-by-step instructions to grow your businesses. And I get it, yes, we need to know the steps to take but there's another part of the equation. Here's an example: I was working with an Esthetician who hired me to help her grow her business. She numbered off each action she was already taking to move toward this goal. She had her bases covered perfectly. But when I asked her how she was feeling about her business, she said that she was frustrated, very nervous, and constantly thinking about what else she should be doing. She had done everything just right to set herself up for success, now she needed to step back, stop thinking so much, and have some fun with it; that was the missing piece for her.

Think about those who are frustrated and worried. Their bodies are closed off and the energy around them is unapproachable. Now picture those who trust that they've got it covered, business is on its way, no worries. Their body language is more confident and their energy is open to attracting business. Follow the steps you need to take to grow your business, but also pay attention to how you feel, because how you feel does show. Have faith that the clients will come.

The words you speak are very powerful. This is for real!! If you spend your time talking about how slow business is, it will continue to be slow. If you spend your time talking about how scared you are about money, you will continue to have money issues to be scared about. Seriously....it's that simple. You get what you talk about. Let me repeat that...you get what you talk about. When I purchased my first skin care center back in 1990, it was slow! I mean really slow! But anytime a client would come in and ask me how I was doing, the answer was always "fabulous, business is booming and I couldn't be happier". Even if it was Thursday and she was my first client of the week. I was still fabulous. Don't tell it like it is, tell it like you want it to be. Let me repeat this one also…don't tell it like it is, tell it like you want it to be. If you were a fly on the wall at my house, you would think that my husband and I had lost our minds. A few years ago, we started talking continuously about how we wanted things to be. Each day, we would sit and have a conversation about the beautiful big home we live in, the fabulous parties we have our friends over for, the cars we have in our 3-car garage, how the training business is booming, and how I am a household name to all my fellow Estheticians.

We talked in the present, like we were living all of that right then and there. Well, we lived in a 950 square-foot townhouse with a view of the townhouse across the walkway. For a short while, we had only one car. We definitely didn't have any parties because there was barely enough space for the two of us and our two dogs, and barely anyone in the esthetic world knew who Shelley Hancock was, but we kept talking every day. Today, we live in a home big enough to have a fabulous party. We've got two nice cars and while I'm not a household name yet, many more Estheticians know who I am. All of this was because we told our story like we wanted it to be, not like it was.

I had only been an Esthetician a year and a half when I purchased that first skin care center and I became super successful. Why? First, my passion to become successful was huge and second, I was present. Emotionally and physically. I went to my Center every single day whether I had a client or not. I wanted to be there just in case the phone rang or someone happened to stop by. I wanted to be there to show the universe that I was serious about being successful. Cell phones weren't really around back then so I didn't have the option of being at the mall and still answering a phone call. I cannot tell you how many times I have called an Esthetician who has left me a message and when she picks up the phone, I can clearly tell she's lunching with the girls or shopping or doing something that has nothing at all to do with her business. Her mind is not focused on business. I personally feel like this has been part of the downfall for some business owners. Their energy is scattered. There is no complete focus on business during business hours.

Let's chat about your phone voice. It is your chance to make a good first impression and if it's not a good one, you've lost them at the get go. Does your voice sound monotone or non-interested? Are you talking so loud that they must hold the phone away from their ears or too soft so they can barely hear you? Do you sound depressed, like the weight of the world is on your shoulders? Are you speaking so fast that it's too hard to understand you? Sometimes, I'll get a message from an Esthetician who wants me to call her back and when she says her phone number she goes on warp speed! If a client must listen to your message three times to try to understand you, that is not a good thing. I'm guessing they may get frustrated, hang up, and go elsewhere. So, be very aware of your phone voice.

Listening is extremely important. Do you really listen to your clients or do you prefer the sound of your own voice? People love to feel like they are being heard. Ask your clients questions about their needs and then stop and listen to what they have to say. Be present. Don't be thinking about what you are going to say back to them. Really listen. To create that relationship, that strong bond that keeps those clients coming back, you must learn how to stop and listen.

We become psychologists in the treatment room, don't we? Our clients lay down on that treatment bed and boy, do the stories just come spilling out. Our clients come to us to get away from the world for an hour. Keep your conversations light or better yet, take your cue from the client. If she's quiet, you should be quiet also. If she's chatty, let her chat away. But if it's negative subject matter, steer her toward the positive. Instead of helping her go deeper into the muck, ask her questions about how she would like things to be. Don't feed into negativity by encouraging her or agreeing with her. Politely steer her in another direction. Get her thinking about the positive aspects of life. She may not thank you right away, but you are doing her a big favor. She's probably so used to being in the muck, that if you take her out of the muck, she'll leave feeling so good (she probably won't even really know why she's feeling so good) that she will want to come back for more!

Okay, very last thing and it's a big one. Gratitude. It is so powerful. Try spending more time each day being thankful for what you do have and no time whatsoever complaining about what you don't have. The more gratitude you show, the more things you will get to be grateful for. If you only have one client today and it's just a quick lip wax, do not complain about having just one client; be grateful for this client. Say a silent thank you for her business, a thank you for the income. Pretty soon, you'll have two and then three and then four clients to be thankful for. Try it, it really works!

So, take a moment and check in to see where you may be slightly veering off track in your career. There could be just one little thing you can tweak and it ends up making all the difference in the world to how successful you become. Challenge yourself and see how things change.

About Shelley Hancock

Shelley Hancock, (a.k.a 'The Gadget Gal'), is one of the most trusted esthetic advisors of our time and Founder of Shelley Hancock Consulting, an organization dedicated to helping estheticians increase their profits. After owning a successful skin care center for 29 years, Hancock expanded her focus so she could provide a deeper level of service to fellow estheticians. Through hands-on training, workshops and private consultations, she has now connected 1000s of beauty business owners with esthetic equipment that attracts a higher level client and helps build a more successful practice. "Most retailers think the relationship ends with purchase," explains Hancock. "I view it as just the beginning".

When she's not teaching, training, coaching or working with clients, you will find her recording her radio program for Voice America.

Contact Shelley Today!
Website: http://www.ShelleyHancock.com
Email: contactme@shelleyhancock.com

Notes

Made in the USA
Lexington, KY
15 December 2019